# Eat Wholefoods
# And Take
# Supplements

## The Ultimate Lifestyle Guide
## For Health, Nutrition And Wellness

# Also By Brian B Jacques

His very popular Series of Mini-Health Books includes:

- An Easy Way To Understand Eczema and Psoriasis
- An Easy Way To Understand Stress and Depression
- Amino Acids & Enzymes—What Are They & Why Do You Need Them
- An Easy Way To Understand Vitamins and Minerals
- An Easy Way To Understand Crohn's Disease and IBD
- An Easy Way To Understand Body Building For Men And Women
- An Easy Way To Understand Parasites, Worms, Candida, Constipation & Detoxing
- An Easy Way To Understand Alzheimer's Disease
- An Easy Way To Understand Herpes
- An Easy Way To Understand Parkinson's Disease
- An Easy Way To Understand Autism
- An Easy Way To Understand Fibromyalgia
- The Little A–Z Dictionary of Herbal Remedies
- Effective Methods To Stop Smoking
- The Magic Of Vitamins & Minerals
- An Easy Way To Understand Your Body Systems
- An Easy Way To Understand Erectile Dysfunction
- An Easy Way To Understand Heart Disease, High Blood Pressure & Stroke
- An Easy Way To Understand Detoxing For Men & Women
- How To Lose Weight After 40
- How To Lose Weight And Maintain Your Ideal Weight Permanently
- Herbs For Healing—101 Herbal Remedies—What Are They, What Are They Used For

All these books are also available as Kindle Editions (available from the Kindle Store on Amazon.com, and other countries Amazon sites where the Kindle platform is supported.) Many of these books are also available for the Barnes and Noble "Nook".In addition, all these titles will shortly be available as print editions from the Amazon website.

# Eat Wholefoods
# And Take
# Supplements
## The Ultimate Lifestyle Guide
## For Health Nutrition And Wellness

**Brian B Jacques.**

**Part of a Series of Mini Health Books**

Wisdom For Life Media

**Publisher: Wisdom For Life Media**

While they have made every effort to verify the information provided in this book, neither the author nor the publisher assumes any responsibility for errors in, omissions from, or different interpretation of the subject matter.

The information herein may be subject to varying laws, regulations, and practices in different areas, states and countries. The purchaser or reader assumes all responsibility for use of the information.

All information included within this book is for educational purposes only. The author and publishers do not attempt to diagnose or treat any medical conditions, be it to do with health, diet or exercise.

If you consider that you have any kind of medical condition, then, you should consult a qualified medical practitioner or doctor before starting any vitamin and/or mineral program or supplement regime, exercise or health training program or diet suggested in this book.

This book is not intended for anyone under the age of 18 years, nor is it intended for breast feeding or pregnant women, underweight people or anyone with eating disorders or a health condition that requires special diets or medical treatment.

The author and publishers disclaim any liability for any loss however caused by anyone using the information contained in this book.

**Images**

"Choose My Plate" Copyright USDA Center for Nutrition Policy and Promotion. www.choosemyplate.gov

All other images are either copyright the author or are used under the terms of a royalty free license.

ISBN - 13: 978-1508504429

ISBN - 10: 1508504423

Printed and published in the United States of America

*"Education is the kindling of a flame, not the filling of a vessel."*—Socrates

# Contents

# Acknowledgment

To the many people I have come into contact with
throughout my life, whose belief in me has made
everything possible and worthwhile.

# Part One
## Whole Foods Verses Processed Foods

# Chapter 1

## Whole Foods Defined

Whole foods are best defined as foods that are eaten in their natural state without any processing or refining. They do not contain any additives such as preservatives, chemicals, salt, sugar or fat.

In most cases, the term whole foods usually refers to vegetables, fruits, and whole grains, but, protein can also be defined as a whole food if it does not include any processing. For example, a plain chicken breast as opposed to chicken nuggets, or grilled fish as opposed to fish sticks.

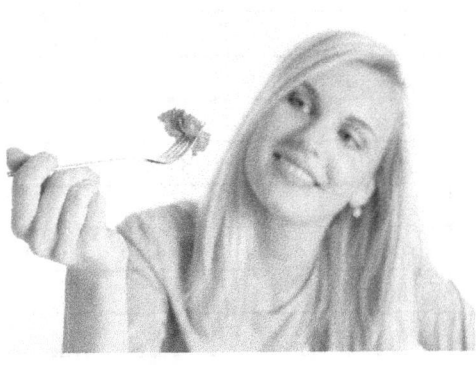

It should not be assumed that whole foods are organic. Some whole foods can be organic, but they are not automatically classified as such.

In addition, very few countries have an organic certification program like they do in the US and UK.

When a whole food is processed it removes all the vital nutrients that the whole food contained in its original state. As a result, there is little contribution to wellness which would have been the case if the food had been eaten in its natural form.

Good examples include: white bread, white rice, pasta, and other grain foods that are refined. When the grain is processed, valuable nutrients are removed such as fiber when the coat of the grain and the bran are removed. And that is not all, as you can see in the following table important minerals are also lost as well. All minerals have to be obtained from the diet; the body does not manufacture any minerals itself.

| Percentage of Minerals Lost Through Food Processing | | | |
|---|---|---|---|
| | White Flour | Sugar Refining | Rice Polishing |
| Chromium | 98% | 78% | 86% |
| Manganese | 92% | 54% | 75% |
| Zinc | 95% | 88% | 89% |

| Percentage of Minerals Lost Through Refining Flour | | | |
|---|---|---|---|
| Calcium | 60% | Molybdenum | 48% |
| Chromium | 98% | Phosphorus | 71% |
| Cobalt | 89% | Potassium | 77% |
| Copper | 68% | Selenium | 16% |
| Iron | 76% | Sodium | 78% |
| Magnesium | 85% | Zinc | 78% |
| Manganese | 86% | | |

In addition, processing whole foods often adds additional unnecessary ingredients including sugar and fat

Whole foods are dense in essential nutrients whilst processed (refined) foods are energy dense.

### So what is the difference?

Foods that are dense in essential nutrients provide vital nutrition the body needs, such as vitamins, minerals, fiber and antioxidants without added sugar and fat. By comparison, energy dense foods are often high in empty calories that provide little or no nutrition.

Ideally a whole food is one ingredient, for example, an apple, chicken breast, baked sweet potato wedges, cucumber and steel-cut oatmeal.

While we may prepare and cook these ingredients in combination to make a multi ingredient dish, the foods themselves maintain their whole integrity because they are not altered.

For example: A grilled chicken breast eaten with baked sweet potato wedges on the side is a whole food meal, but, a fried chicken breast with a side of French fries is a processed meal.

Another Example: A baked potato is a whole food, potato chips is a processed food.

**What Is Wholesome Eating**

Wholesome eating as its name suggests, is a term that refers to following a diet that is exclusively comprised of whole foods.

When you eat wholesome foods, your diet comprises foods eaten in their natural state without added: fats, sugars, high fructose corn syrup, preservatives, artificial flavors, colors, textures or any other chemicals.

Eating wholesome also means avoiding "fake foods" or those chemically created foods that have no real food in them.

# Chapter 2

## What Are Processed Foods

Processed foods did not exist during the times of early man and really before the industrial revolution. There were no aisles filled with ready prepared meals, fruit pies or cookies. There was no drive thru fast food outlets where French fries, chicken nuggets and chili cheese fries are available.

All food was obtained from natural sources, fruits and vegetables grown from plants and trees, meat from hunting and the human diet was eaten in its natural state. It was often cooked over an open flame or an early version of the modern stove or oven which ran on wood.

Looking at the pie charts, you will see that the average diet is nothing like it used to be centuries ago. It has shifted, particularly in the past forty years or so to a more high (saturated) fat and sugar diet.

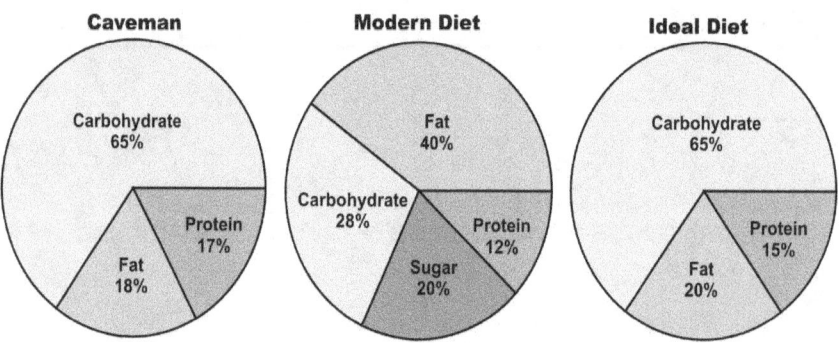

A lot of this has come about through clever marketing and the "now society" in which we live, where everything has to be quick and easy. And everything is done on the run, with no time to sit down and eat a meal properly. How often do you see people at lunchtime, walking down the street eating their lunch as they walk along, or ordering their lunch at a drive thru facility in a fast food outlet, then the lunch is eaten as the person drives along. This practice is hardly conducive to good digestion and good health.

While some form of processing is  involved in all foods we eat—unless we stick with a completely 100% raw food diet, for example, cooking is a form of processing or grinding steak into a hamburger, that is not the definition of processing I am referring to here.

There is a distinct difference between mechanical and chemical processing.

Chemical processing by definition means that food has been altered from its original state and then becomes refined with additives, preservatives and other ingredients that make it "highly processed". This has the effect of turning a one ingredient food item into a 3, 4 or more ingredient dish. Refined is another term used for highly processed food.

In summary, any food that is not eaten in its original "whole state" is then processed or refined. For example, a peach is a whole food, peach pie is not.

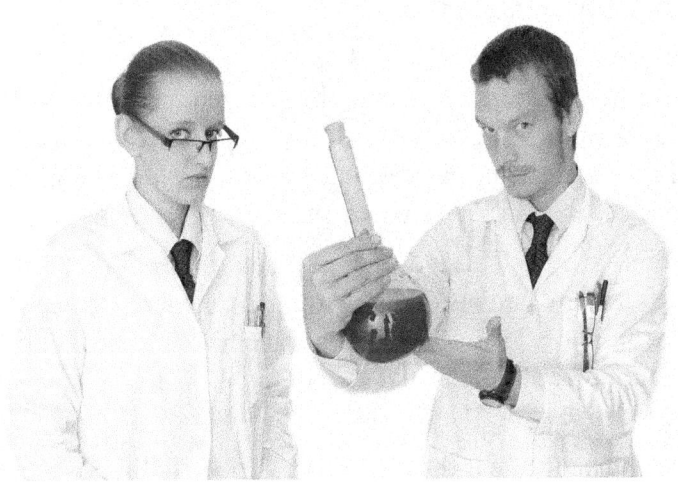

## Chapter 3

## Why Are Vitamins and Minerals So Important?

Vitamins and minerals are as vital in keeping the body going as the fuel, lubricating oil and water in our cars. Without them, we'd simply stop functioning. But how vital are they? Do most of us get the right ones in the right quantities? Let's take a look.

There's been a debate raging for years about whether a proper balanced diet gives you all that you need in terms of vitamins and minerals or whether you need to take supplements to top up your levels. Some doctors are convinced that if you eat properly there's no need for you to take vitamin and mineral supplements, although often they're important for people who are ill, or pregnant women. Others disagree, saying that supplements are essential to make sure we're properly nourished.

So, what is a balanced diet? And is it suitable for everyone? The answer is no, it is not. The human body is made up of approximately 63 percent water, 22 percent protein, 13 percent fat, and 2 percent vitamins and minerals. Everything—every molecule comes from the food you eat and the water you drink.

Someone who is elderly needs a totally different diet to say a top flight sportsman who needs extra amounts of energy to keep his body in peak condition. Likewise, someone who has a physically demanding job would need different dietary requirements to say someone who leads a sedentary lifestyle.

It is important to eat the best quality food that you can afford, in the correct quantities in order to get the maximum energy, health and freedom from disease. But when we look at the "best quality food", we have to take into account the growing methods of crops, where chemical fertilizers and pesticides are the norm and animal husbandry, where the use of antibiotics and growth promoters are used extensively. All these factors have dramatically changed the quality of our food over the years.

In years gone by, it was common practice for a farmer to exercise crop rotation, and to let certain fields lie fallow for a season in order for them to rest and regenerate themselves. Not anymore! Now as soon as one crop is harvested, the field is ploughed over again, it is them treated with chemical pest control agents and nutrients and a new crop is sown.

Many people, of course, eat properly and take the occasional supplement as well, particularly if they've been ill or under the weather. If you do take supplements, make sure you're well informed about exactly what they do, and only take natural ones—not synthetic ones.

We will look at why vitamins and minerals are vital for good health and whether you can benefit from a few extra ones in part two of this book.

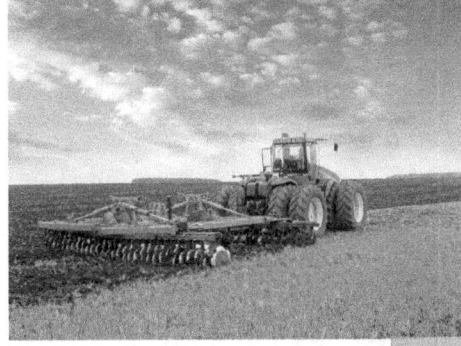

## Chapter 4

## 40 Examples of Whole Food Compared to Processed Food

1. Strawberries compared to strawberry pop tarts

2. Raspberries compared to raspberry pop tarts

3. Fresh berries compared to fruit filled Danish or jelly filled donuts

4. Whole fruit bars compared to cereal bars

5. Butter compared to margarine

6. Whole peaches compared to peach cocktail

7. Brown or wild rice compared to white rice

8. Pinto beans compared to canned refried beans

9. Whole grain bread compared to white bread

10. Whole fruit compared to fruit roll ups

11. Oranges or 100% pure orange juice compared to orange drinks or orange concentrate

12. Grilled or raw onions compared to Funyuns

13. Tomatoes compared to canned tomato soup

14. Corn on the cob compared to corn chips or corn flakes

15. Baked potato compared to potato chips

16. Baked potato compared to French fries

17. Raw or grilled onions compared to onion rings

18. Grilled fish fillet compared to fish sticks

19. Grilled chicken breast compared to chicken nuggets or coated fried chicken

20. Whole vegetables compared to veggie chips

21. Grilled pork chop compared to bacon

22. Slice of roast beef or turkey right from the roast or bird compared to spam, hot dogs and lunch meats

23. Raw almonds and other nuts compared to chocolate covered, smoked or flavored nut products

24. Grilled shrimp compared to fried shrimp

25. Raw spinach compared to cream of spinach

26. Corn on the cob compared to canned creamed corn

27. Grapes compared to raisins

28. Whole berries compared to preserves

29. Whole berries compared to berry ice cream toppings

30. Bananas compared to banana chips

31. Bananas compared to frozen banana desserts

32. White tortillas compared to whole grain tortillas

33. Whole wheat, barley, almond, rye or any whole grain flour compared to white refined flour

34. 60% + cacao dark chocolate compared to Snickers, Kit Kat or other chocolate candy bars

35. Black coffee compared to Mocha Frappuccino

36. Food you can pronounce compared to any food that is or has unpronounceable ingredients

37. Block of Mozzarella cheese compared to American cheese slices, Velveeta, bagged shredded cheese, or nacho cheese sauce

38. Full fat yogurt, cottage cheese or sour cream compared to nonfat or low fat (it takes processing to remove fat from these dairy products)

39. Plain yogurt compared to flavored or fruit at the bottom yogurt products

40. Non-homogenized milk and dairy products compared to their homogenized counterparts

# Chapter 5

## Processed Foods Can Be Harmful

### Additives and Artificial Ingredients

Often times looking at a processed food ingredient list, you feel like you need a degree in chemistry—if you have a degree in chemistry, then perhaps you can educate the rest of us!

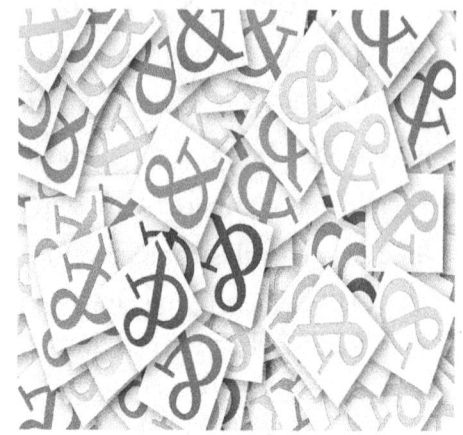

Processed food ingredient lists often contain words that no one can pronounce which signals added ingredients that the body does not need.

Think about it, in order for any type of processed food to have any kind of shelf life a preservative has to be used. This is then followed by an artificial flavor, because, unless the food is whole—and there are no processed foods in nature—it has to get its flavor from somewhere.

These additive ingredients are all chemicals or chemically created, they are not real whole food.

### Highly Processed Foods Contain These Extras

Here are just a few of the added ingredients in processed foods.

INGREDIENTS: ENRICHED WHEAT FLOUR (WHEAT FLOUR, NIACIN, REDUCED IRON, THIAMIN MONONITRATE [VITAMIN B1], RIBOFLAVIN [VITAMIN B2], FOLIC ACID), HIGH FRUCTOSE CORN SYRUP, ONIONS*, SALT, CONTAINS LESS THAN 2% OF HYDROLYZED SOY PROTEIN, YEAST, PARTIALLY HYDROGENATED SOYBEAN AND/OR COTTONSEED OIL, COOKED CHICKEN AND CHICKEN BROTH, CELERY*, MONOSODIUM GLUTAMATE, PARSLEY*, SPICE, MALTODEXTRIN, POTASSIUM CHLORIDE, SUGAR, TURMERIC, DISODIUM GUANYLATE, DISODIUM INOSINATE, NATURAL FLAVOR, WITH BHA, BHT, PROPYL GALLATE, AND CITRIC ACID AS PRESERVATIVES.

- Coloring—chemicals that give food a certain color
- Preservatives—to extend shelf life
- Artificial flavoring—chemicals to add a specific flavor or a flavor blend. This can include a mix of many different chemicals
- Texturant—chemicals that provide a certain type of texture to a processed food

## High Unhealthy Fat Content

Processed foods often contain high amounts of unhealthy fats.

Hydrogenated fat in processed foods causes one of the biggest problems as the processing converts them into trans-fat. The Mayo Clinic calls trans-fat "double trouble for your heart health". Trans fats have the effect of raising your LDL (bad cholesterol) and lowering your HDL (good cholesterol), This is one of the worst type of fat for the human body as it is a major player in 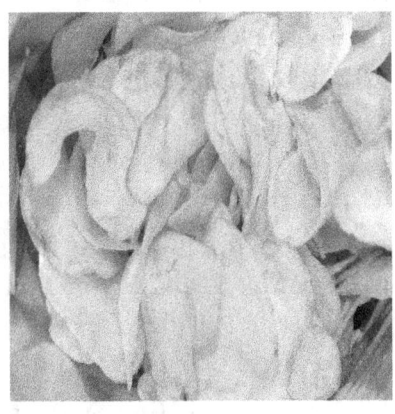 increasing risks for heart disease and high cholesterol.

So what is trans-fat? Various meat and dairy products contain a small amount of naturally occurring trans-fat. However, the majority of trans-fat is formed in an industrial process that adds hydrogen to vegetable oil. This process has the effect of solidifying the oil at room temperature. This partially hydrogenated oil creates a longer shelf life in foods which means they do not spoil as easily.

In fact, some restaurants often use partially hydrogenated vegetable oil in their deep fryers as the oil does not need to be changed as often as non-hydrogenated oil.

The manufactured form of trans-fat called partially hydrogenated oil is found in a wide variety of foods such as:

**Baked goods** (the majority of cakes, cookies, pie crusts and crackers).

**Snacks** (Most potato, corn and tortilla chips as well as popcorn).

**Fried foods** (French fries, doughnuts and fried chicken).

**Refrigerator dough** (canned biscuits, cinnamon rolls, frozen pizza crusts).

**Creamer and margarine** (Nondairy coffee creamer and stick margarines).

And what about those products you see in the shops that say "No Trans-Fat"? Well, in the United States if a food contains less than 0.5

grams of trans-fat per serving, then it can be labeled "0 grams trans-fat". Bear in mind this "undeclared" trans-fat can add up really quickly, especially if you eat multiple serving of various foods that contain this "hidden" 0.5 grams of trans-fat.

So become an avid label reader. Check the foods ingredient list. Look for "partially hydrogenated vegetable oil". If you see this, then the food contains a certain amount of trans-fat possibly below the 0.5 grams declaration level. So beware!

However, it is not all bad news. There are healthy "real" fats such as butter, olive oil, and coconut oil which provide the body with healthy fats and because they are not processed, they are considered as whole foods—unlike their unfriendly relatives.

## High Sugar and High Fructose Corn Syrup Content

Many processed foods contain copious amounts of added sugar and high fructose corn syrup which is harmful for your health.

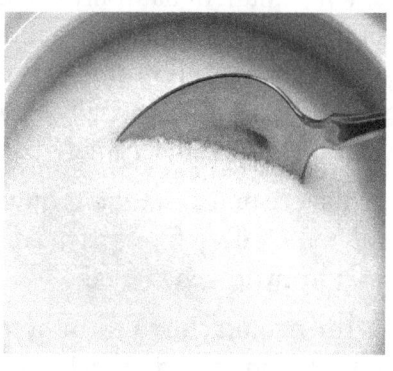

Sugar in particular is a highly addictive substance. It can have a profound effect on blood sugar levels, and is in effect an empty calorie food. If it is consumed in excessive amounts it can cause feelings of euphoria that mimic illegal drugs. So a sugar dependency can develop to maintain that "high" with the result that over indulgence occurs.

Empty calories in sugar are also a contributory factor in weight gain and obesity as many studies have shown that sugar has a significant effect on the body's metabolism.

If sugar is consumed in excess it can eventually lead to insulin resistance, high cholesterol and also increased fat accumulation in the liver and the belly. It can also lead to heart disease, and Type 2 Diabetes.

## Overindulgence and Addiction

Processed foods stimulate the various pleasure centers in the brain and as a result, an increased desire for these types of foods can develop so we over eat on them. Consider donuts, candy, French fries and soda, can you eat just one?

These foods have been engineered to be rewarding to the brain and bring us pleasure, as opposed to natural whole foods that are intended for sustenance.

Once we are hooked on these foods as a result of their hyper-rewarding nature we crave them, need them and our appetites gravitate towards the sweet, fatty and salty concoctions that in reality—hold very little nutritional value.

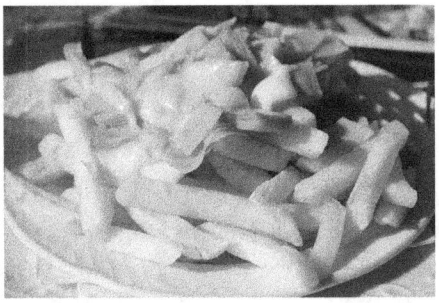

Food addiction is a serious health condition that can have a really negative effect on people's health. Unfortunately no one becomes addicted to lettuce or apples. Food addiction always revolves around junk food, sweet and unhealthy fatty and salty foods because, as mentioned above, these foods activate pleasure and reward centers in the brain just like heroin and cocaine.

Processed foods typically tend to overpower any food source found in nature, but, an individual can always adjust their food habits and change their food tastes.

## Lack of Nutrients

It is well known that lowering as well as regulating calorie intake is the best way to pursue healthy weight management. However, not all calories are created equal.

Kale, chicken breast and apples are all nutrient rich whole foods that provide an excellent source of nutrition calorie for calorie. When we eat them our bodies use the nutrients to thrive and boost our health.

Processed foods by comparison are lacking in nutrients and so they provide empty calorie foods that the body just stores as fat, and as a result, they do not benefit the body in any way.

They are lacking in macronutrients, like protein, healthy fats and complex carbohydrates, and they also lack micronutrients such as vitamins, minerals and fiber.

Natural whole foods that come from plants and animals contain a large amount of trace nutrients, many of which have not yet been identified, but it is known that they benefit the human body.

And to date, there is no way to mimic these vital natural nutrients in a lab.

## Reduced Thermic Effect of Food

What is the Thermic Effect of Food (TEF)? It is a term used to measure the energy expenditure (metabolism) after eating particular foods, specifically it totals approximately 10% of the metabolic rate in the average person.

According to a study published in the journal *Food & Nutrition Research* in 2010, the metabolic rate of 17 men and women was compared after they ate a processed meal and a whole food meal. Those who had a multi grain bread cheddar cheese sandwich burned twice as many calories as those who ate a white bread American cheese sandwich.

So, the conclusion was that whole foods are burned more efficiently by the body than processed foods, which supports the healthy weight management concept of "calories in equates to calories out."

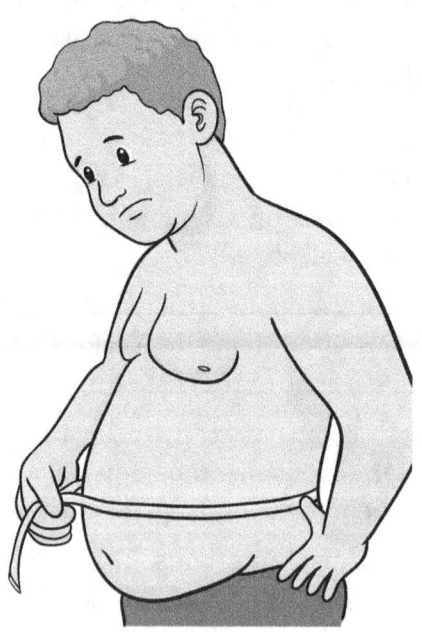

# Chapter 6

# Characteristics of the Healthiest Foods

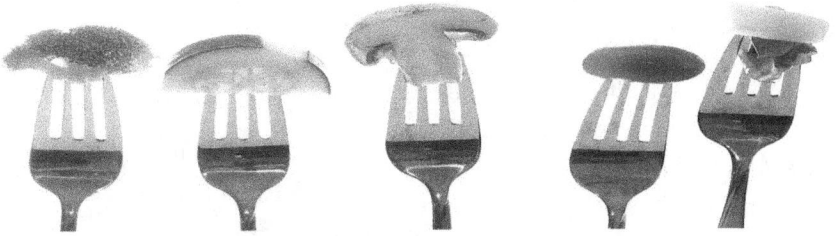

There are literally thousands of foods in existence. Most of these foods provide a source of essential nutrients that humans need to incorporate into their diet in order to be healthy. The world's healthiest foods have very specific characteristics.

## Full of Nutrients

The healthiest foods in the world are sources of numerous nutrients that play a key role in creating and preserving your health. These foods possess a higher nutritional value than any other food.

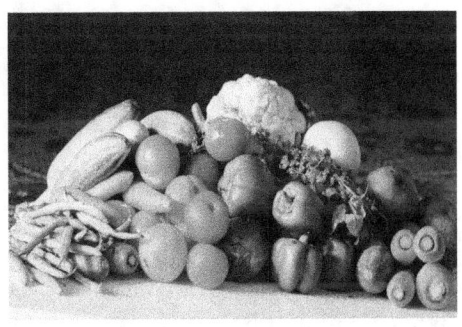

Basically, they contain a very high proportion of nutrients and a very low proportion of calories. The world's healthiest foods provide you with all of the nutrients that you need in order to enjoy outstanding health. These nutrients are vitamins, minerals, antioxidants, protein, fiber, phytonutrients, fatty acids, and enzymes along with the lowest possible amount of calories.

The best way to define whole foods is to say that they are foods that contain all of the nutrients that they can possibly contain, in addition, they are unprocessed and they are free of artificial ingredients.

## They Are Easily Recognizable

The world's healthiest foods are staples of the diet that everyone knows and can recognize. They include: fruits, vegetables, whole grains, meat and fish. These are all examples of the world's healthiest foods.

### They Are Easy To Obtain

The world's healthiest foods are readily available in any food market in any part of the world.

### They Are Affordable

The world's healthiest foods are inexpensive to buy. They are cheapest when purchased locally and in season, which means they will be of the best quality.

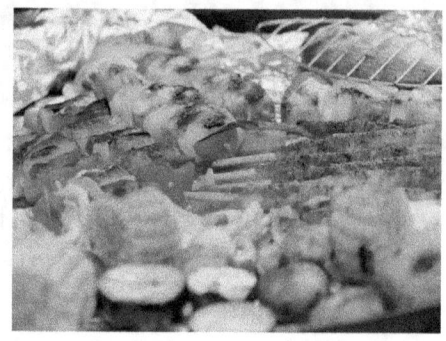

### They Are Delicious To Eat

Fortunately, the world's healthiest foods are in many cases the most delicious foods in the world, especially once you do a body detox to purge the highly addictive processed foods that are loaded with sugar and unhealthy fats from your system.

### They Improve Health

Eating the world's healthiest foods provides many health benefits. Ideally, you should eat them when they are fresh and organically grown in order for your body systems to derive the maximum benefits from them.

### They Help Prevent Disease

The healthiest foods, such as, whole foods that include, fruits, vegetables and whole grains contain essential disease preventing antioxidants which help neutralize the damaging effects of free radicals in the body. Everyone has free radicals—they are unavoidable. They are derived from the air you breathe, and from the food you eat. The body also generates free radicals as a metabolic by-product of mineral absorption. So, by consuming antioxidants, you will be decreasing your risk of developing various cancers, chronic diseases, as well as aging healthily and enjoying high energy levels.

You will also be helping prevent the onset of other illnesses, such as cardiovascular disease, arthritis, asthma and bronchitis.

Furthermore, eating healthy foods improves your vision. This is because antioxidants help prevent the development of cataracts.

Cataracts impair your vision, which is caused by the eye's lens becoming cloudy. Consequently, by incorporating antioxidants in your diet, you are helping to preserve your vision.

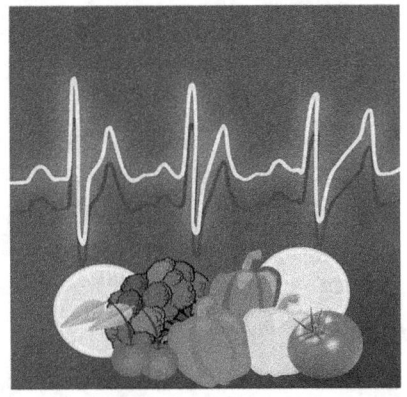

## They Contain Phytoestrogens

Phyto- is from the Greek word phyton meaning plant. A phytoestrogen is a naturally-occurring plant nutrient that exerts an estrogen-like action on the body. Phytoestrogens exist in plant-based foods, such as soy beans, berries and flaxseeds. Research indicates that people who consume large amounts of phytoestrogens are less likely to suffer from breast cancer, ovarian cancer and endometrial cancer than people who do not consume them.

## They Contain Dietary Fiber

Dietary fiber and resistant starches are to be found in whole grains. Unfortunately, fiber is sadly lacking in the average American diet due to it being high in processed foods which contain excessive amounts of fat, sugar and various additives. Dietary fiber improves digestion and strengthens the lining of the intestinal tract, and aids in the prevention of constipation—another American dietary problem. Dietary fiber also plays a key role in healthy weight management, prevention of heart disease and keeping vital organs healthy.

# Chapter 7

## 7 Benefits of Whole Foods

The U.S. Department of Agriculture (USDA) reports that as many as 1/3rd of the US population do not get sufficient essential nutrients in their diets, including the all-important antioxidants, vitamin C, vitamin A, magnesium and more than 90% of the American population do not get enough fiber and potassium in their diets.

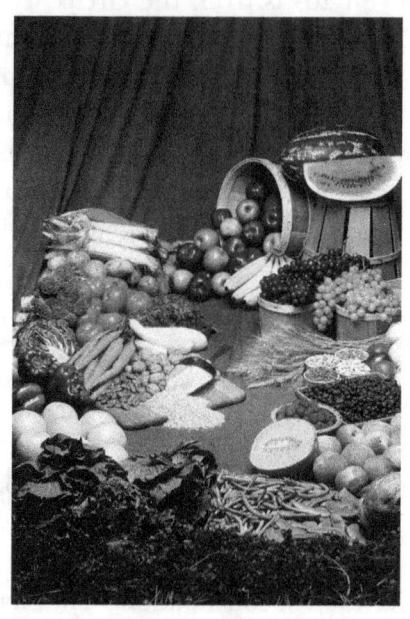

And, if that is not bad enough, the American Institute for Cancer Research (AICR) reports that, the nutrients we lack are some of the most important for heart health, and to prevent major chronic diseases, like, cancer, high blood pressure, and diabetes.

Therefore the solution is really simple—Eat Whole Food—and/or take dietary supplements (see Part Two)!

It is important to understand that a balanced diet filled with plant food along with a dietary supplement program is the best way to ensure a long and healthy life, free of obesity and disease and filled with energy and vitality. Why do I suggest a dietary supplement program as well? As you will read in part two of this book, it can be difficult to get all the nutrients your body requires from the food you eat. Here are some of the reasons why. It is all to do with the way food is grown, harvested, processed, stored and cooked. All of these issues will have a profound effect on how much nutrient value you get out of the food when you eat it. Therefore, a dietary supplement program may be needed to make up for any nutrient shortfall.

### Nutrients For Optimal Health

A diet that comprises whole foods, including, vegetables, fruits, whole grains, legumes, seeds and nuts ensures the human body receives high concentrations of antioxidants, fiber and many important phytochemicals that can protect it from chronic diseases. But this is not always enough. It all depends on your age and lifestyle, as well as the quality of the food you are eating. Therefore, antioxidant supplements such as beta carotene, vitamin C, Zinc, and vitamin E may be worth considering as well.

**Whole Foods Provide**

- Complex micronutrients
- Essential dietary fiber
- Essential antioxidants, including the all-important phytochemicals
- Natural synergy where all the essential nutrients are working together

**Whole Food's Reduce The Risk Of**

- Heart disease
- Various types of cancer
- Type 2 diabetes
- Many other chronic and acute conditions

**Antioxidants**

I have covered the need for antioxidants in more detail in part two. However, here is a "taster" to get you started on this fascinating subject.

Essential antioxidants play a major role in maintaining good health and preventing chronic disease. Various studies have shown that antioxidants, which, include, vitamin C, vitamin A, lycopene, phytochemicals, and carotenoids lower the risk of developing various types of cancer and other chronic diseases.

Free radicals damage human cells through a process called oxidation and as a result can cause several chronic illnesses.

Antioxidants boost immunity, protect against free radicals, and lower risks of developing cancer and heart disease.

Largely plant based foods are those highest in essential antioxidants, this includes, all deep colored fresh fruits and vegetables—nature's whole foods.

## Phytochemicals

Researchers have identified many biologically active components found in plants called phytochemicals, including:

- Lycopene, which, is a red colored carotenoid mainly found in tomatoes
- Anthocyanins that give blueberries their blue color
- Pterostilbene that works to break down fat and cholesterol (mainly found in blueberries and dark purple grapes used in wines, like Pinot Noir)

Phytochemicals play an important role in protecting body cells from free radical damage and foreign body mutations as a result of environmental risk factors. And, the only way to get them into your body is to eat plant foods which contain them in a whole food form.

## Carotenoids

There are more than 600 antioxidants called carotenoids that are found in plant based foods, some of the more important ones are lycopene (important for prostate health), lutein (for vision) and beta-carotene that help to fight cell damage from free radicals. They also help reduce the risk of:

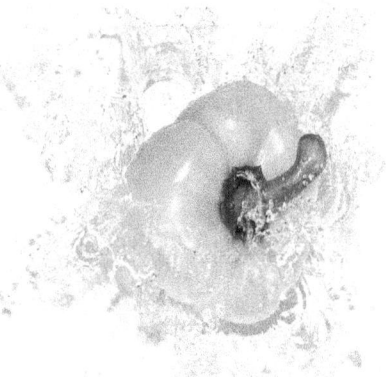

- Prostate cancer
- Cancers of the stomach, mouth, colon, esophagus and rectum

Amongst other body functions, carotenoids are important for eye health. They help reduce the risk of developing cataracts as well as macular degeneration.

## Foods High In Carotenoids

Carotenoids are found in orange, green and red vegetables. It is the carotenoid content which gives them their bright colors:

- Carrots
- Pumpkins

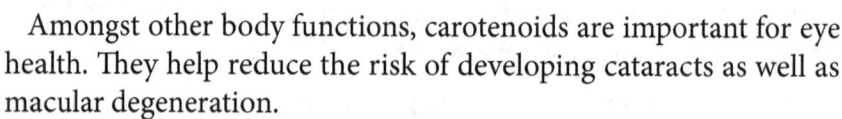

- Squash
- Broccoli
- Orange and yellow peppers
- Sweet potatoes
- Green leafy vegetables
- Tomatoes

## Beta-carotene

Beta-carotene, like all carotenoids, is an antioxidant. Our body does not need beta-carotene specifically, but, what it does need is vitamin A which the body converts beta carotene to as it is needed.

## Benefits Of Vitamin A

- Healthy Skin
- Healthy mucus membranes
- Boosts immunity
- Facilitates eye health

## Foods High In Beta Carotene

- Apricots
- Kale
- Onions
- Peas
- Plums
- Pumpkin
- Spinach
- Asparagus
- Broccoli
- Carrots
- Chinese cabbage
- Chives
- Grapefruit

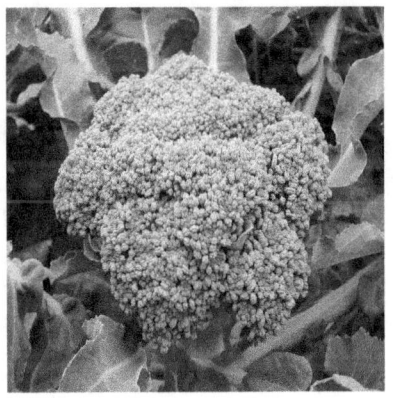

- Herbs/Spices (chili powder, paprika, parsley, oregano)
- Squash
- Sweet potatoes

**Vitamin C**

Vitamin C is a water-soluble antioxidant vitamin that plays a major role in maintaining good health. Vitamin C protects cells from free radical damage, boosts the immune system and assists the body to make collagen, which, is the connective tissue between bones and muscles. When foods containing vitamin C are eaten along with foods rich in iron, it also helps improve iron absorption in the body.

Foods High In Vitamin C:

- Citrus fruits, including, oranges, lemons, grapefruits and tangerines
- Broccoli
- Potatoes
- Papaya
- Strawberries
- Sweet peppers
- Tomatoes
- Mangoes

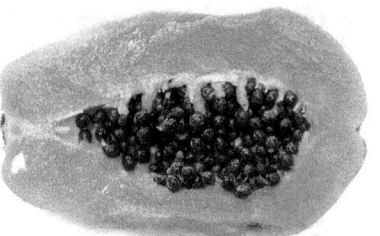

**Good Fats**

A diet that comprises whole foods allows us to get good fats and eliminate the bad ones that are a major cause of high cholesterol and heart disease.

Processed foods are typically loaded with trans-fats and saturated fats that clog heart arteries and play a prominent role in obesity.

On the other hand, whole foods provide good fats, like omega-3 fatty acids that are found in fish, nuts and flax seed, and monounsaturated fat found in various plant sources.

**Fiber**

Fiber is one of the most important nutrients for the human body and supports:

- The digestive system
- Weight loss (fills you up and keeps you satisfied longer)
- The prevention of heart disease
- The prevention of diabetes and assists with stabilizing blood sugars
- Helps keep bowel movements regular which prevents constipation

**Foods High In Fiber (highest amounts):**

- Bran (Oat, Wheat, Corn and Rice bran)
- Beans (Lima, Adzuki, Black, Garbanzo, Lentils, Cranberry Beans, Kidney, Navy, White Beans, Mung, Yellow And Pinto)
- All Berries (Raspberries, Blueberries, Currants, Boysenberries, Gooseberries, Loganberries, Elderberries, and Blackberries)
- Whole Grains (Amaranth, Barley, Buckwheat, air popped popcorn and Bulgur)
- Peas (Blackeye Peas, Split Peas, Green Peas and Pigeon Peas)
- Dark Green Leafy Vegetables (Spinach, all Greens, and Swiss Chard)
- Brassica Vegetables (Kale, Cauliflower, Kohlrabi, Brussels Sprouts, and Broccoli)
- Nuts And Seeds (Almonds, Pinon Nuts, Flaxseed, Sesame Seeds, Sunflower Seeds and Pumpkin Seeds)
- Sweet Potatoes
- Edamame (a fancy name for boiled green soybeans)
- Fruits (Apples, Guava, Jicama, Pears, Persimmons, Avocado, Prunes, Oranges and Figs have the highest counts)

**Omega-3 & Omega 6 Essential Fatty Acids**

According to the Harvard School of Public Health omega 3 fatty acids help to prevent heart disease, contribute to brain health, assist with blood clotting and can prevent stroke.

Omega-3 essential fatty acids are polyunsaturated fats that are not produced naturally by the body, they, can only be obtained from food.

**Foods Rich In Omega-3 Fatty Acids**

- All cold-water fish, with salmon having the most, along with albacore tuna, mackerel, sardines and herring

- Chia seeds

- Edamame

- Flaxseed Oil

- Walnuts

- Flaxseeds

- Pasture Raised Chicken Eggs

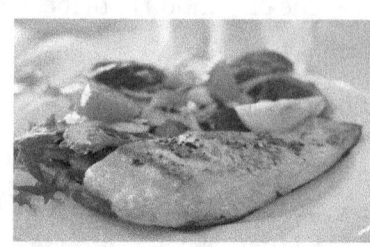

Like Omega 3 Essential Fatty Acids, Omega 6 Essential Fatty Acids (also known as linoleic acid) cannot be made in the body it has to be obtained from the diet. Omega 6 provides support for the brain, bone health, reproductive health, hair growth, and it also helps to regulate your metabolism.

**Main Food sources include**

- Sunflower oil

- Soybean oil

- Avocado oil

- Canola oil

- Flax seed oil

- Palm oil

- Olive oil

- Walnuts

- Safflower seeds

- Brazil nuts

- Sesame seeds

- Pumpkin seeds

- Squash seeds

- Peanuts

- Peanut butter

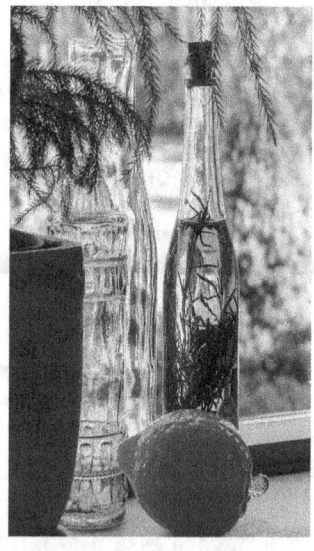

**Balancing Omega 3 and Omega-6 Fats in the Diet**

Because of its high fat and processed content, the Western diet tends to be high in omega 6 essential fatty acids and low in omega 3 Essential Fatty Acids. Omega 6 has a totally different effect to omega 3, in that omega 6 tends to be a cause of inflammation in the body, whilst omega 3 has anti-inflammatory tendencies. I have covered the ideal omega-3 to omega-6 rations in part two of this book on page 94.

Remember the inflammatory consequences I mentioned above. This imbalance can lead to obesity, diabetes, and arthritic conditions.

**The Value of Whole Grains**

A major part of wholesome eating is whole grains. While the fiber value of whole grains is well known, while you may not be aware that they provide so much more.

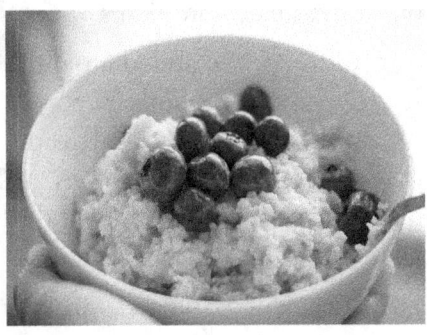

According to, Dr. Simin Liu, a researcher and professor of epidemiology at the University of California-Los Angeles (UCLA), whole grains contain an abundance of vitamins, minerals and phytochemicals that provide substantial health benefits that are far greater than that of dietary fiber.

**These Include**

- Lowering the risk of Type 2 Diabetes and lowering blood glucose levels and insulin after meals.

- Improving cholesterol levels.

- Reducing visceral adipose tissue, which, is a type of unhealthy fat that is deposited between the body's major organs and the abdominal muscles, aka belly fat. A recent study found that excess belly fat is especially harmful and can significantly shorten the life span of both men and women.

**No Additives**

One of the biggest problems with processed foods is not what is missed out, meaning essential nutrients, but, also the hazard of what is included.

The refining process leads to the addition of many additives, in the form of preservatives, coloring, and artificial flavors that are chemically created. The names of many of these ingredients are impossible to pronounce. But, while many individuals are concerned about ingesting these chemical additives, of more impact to human health are the other additives, such as, salt, trans-fat, saturated fat and sugar.

Many medical professionals are concerned about the high consumption of salt in our diets that can lead to high blood pressure (hypertension) and numerous other health problems.

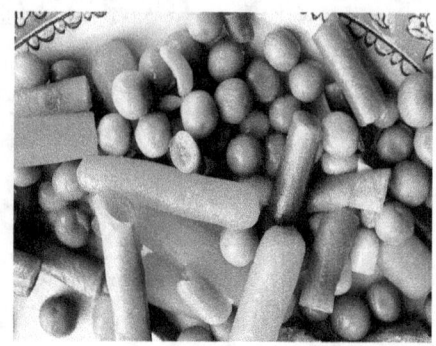

In addition, the added fat and sugar in processed foods increases calories in food which can lead to obesity and being overweight. This in turn leads to major health problems and higher rates of death from heart disease, and Type 2 Diabetes.

On the flip side, wholesome eating where a diet is filled with whole foods allows us to get nutrient dense calories that supply the body with the essential elements it needs which has the added benefit of promoting healthy weight management.

High fiber vegetables and fruits fill you up without the added calories and weight gain.

A diet which is rich in whole foods that includes, fresh fish, lean proteins, green and colored vegetables, whole grains, seeds, nuts, soy protein, natural organic dairy and healthy fats, like olive oil, is your best option to not only help prevent chronic diseases, but, to help you feel and look your absolute best.

### No Counting Required

One of the main benefits of wholesome eating is that you never have to worry about counting anything, including, calories, carbohydrates, fat or sodium intake.

- You don't need gadgets or complicated meal plans
- It is not necessary to buy diet books

- It is not necessary to join online weight loss programs

- You don't have to cope with a restrictive diet

- All you need to do is eat wholesome food—it is that simple

## Weight Control

One of the greatest advantages of wholesome eating is being able to maintain a healthy weight management program that requires no costly diets, buying in special foods or having to plan and prepare complex meals.

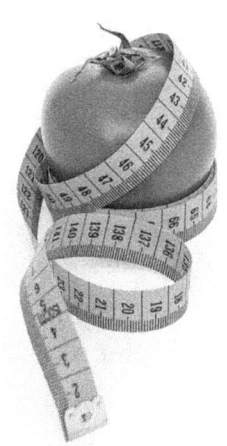

By simply eating food in its natural state you can lose weight and maintain it for life.

According to Texas Tech University Health Sciences Center, eating wholesome foods also provides special benefits for the obese, and those who have high blood pressure, high cholesterol and glucose intolerance.

With whole food being real food, and because it is naturally full of nutrients the calories do not turn to fat like in the case of processed junk food that is full of empty calories. Here are just three examples:

- Eating a medium plain baked potato instead of a medium size French fries from a fast food restaurant saves 215 calories!

- Eating 1 cup of plain yogurt with 1 cup of fresh strawberries instead of a strawberry ice cream Sundae saves 219 calories!

- 1 ounce of corn instead of 1 ounce of corn chips saves 73 calories and 6 grams of fat!

Over the long term these empty calories can add up to a significant amount, and even on a daily basis wholesome eating can yield quite a substantial calorie saving, which can lead to a considerable weight loss.

## Stay Full Longer

Whole foods, such as whole grains, fruits and vegetables, are also high in dietary fiber that fills you up and keeps you full longer so you eat less and lose weight.

## Ditch the Cravings

An interesting fact about eating wholesome foods is that you will notice fairly quickly that your out of control food cravings for such things as donuts, cookies or French fries will disappear.

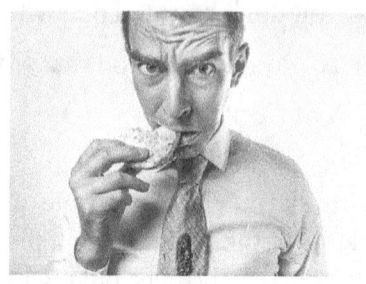

The reason for this is because whole foods balance blood sugar levels, unlike foods which trigger an insulin response, typically candy, which can cause spikes in blood sugar levels which subsequently leads to out of control cravings.

It can take time to get used to eating a wholesome diet and only reaching for whole foods, but, you will get used to it, and it will in all probability become the most important habit you ever develop.

## Cost Effective

Another great bonus to wholesome eating is that it is cheaper than filling your shopping cart with processed foods. In general, the more processed the food, the more costly it is—from a monetary as well as a health standpoint.

## Taste

Last, but by no means least, fresh whole food just plain tastes good. Canned and frozen meals: vegetables, beans, and other products never taste as good as something made fresh with whole ingredients.

Those preservatives and chemicals that are added to extend shelf life affect not only the taste of the food, but the freshness factor as well.

## Real food tastes good!

It is nourishing and so it makes the body feel good and energized, unlike sugary fat filled dishes and products that spike blood sugar levels, which can put your body systems under stress, and cause you to go on a high and then crash and burn, making you feel weighed down, bloated and lethargic.

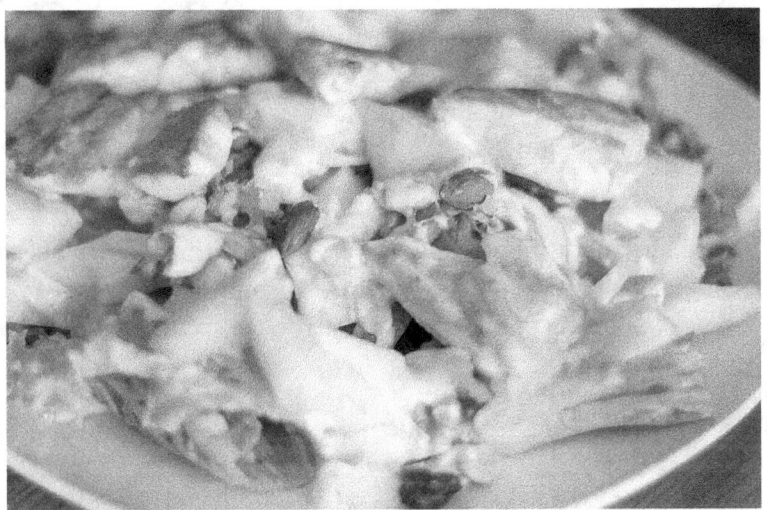

# Chapter 8

## What You Can Eat

What can you eat with a whole food lifestyle?

Any food that is a product of nature, and not of a factory.

Just imagine that the year is 1800 and you can't drive to a fast food outlet for dinner, what would your dinner options be?

### All Fresh Fruits

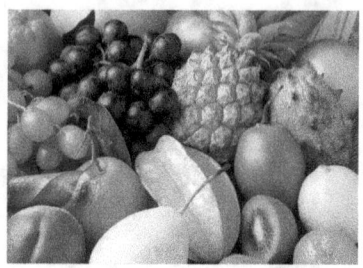

- Organic is best because it is grown without the use of chemicals and pesticides.

- Naturally dried fruit is good. However, it can have a much higher concentrations of sugar than whole fruit.

### All Fresh Vegetables

- Again, organic is best because it is grown without chemicals and pesticides. For a weight management program, be aware of vegetables containing starch, such as carrots, potatoes and corn.

### Dairy And Eggs

Some supporters of a whole food lifestyle advocate against consuming dairy products, but, be mindful that dairy products are your main source of calcium, which along with magnesium and vitamin D (to aid absorption of the minerals) is especially important for women's bone health as a preventative for osteoporosis later in life.

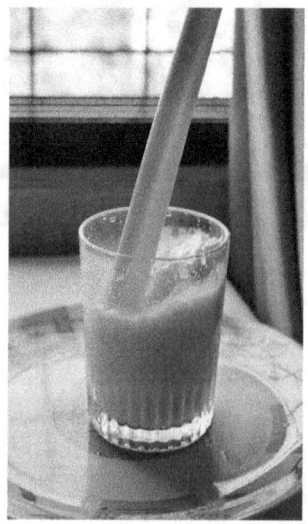

- Raw cows milk, the non-homogenized variety, which is 100% whole, and grass fed is preferable, though harder to get in some states.

- Plain unsweetened yogurt: grass fed and/or organic is best

- Eggs, pasture raised eggs are best.
- Cheese: whole block—not shredded, white cheese has no coloring added, yellow cheeses do. Organic or grass fed variety is best if you can get it.

## 100% Whole Grains

- Millet
- Oats
- Quinoa
- Corn and air popped popcorn (not microwaveable products)
- Rye

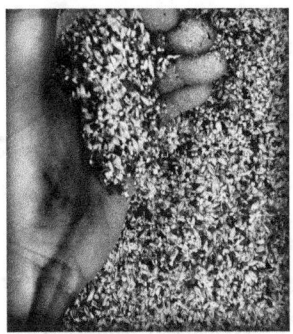

- Whole wheat
- Barley
- Brown rice
- Buckwheat
- Wild Rice

## Poultry & Meats

Grass fed and pasture raised is preferable, here are a few examples.

- Beef
- Chicken

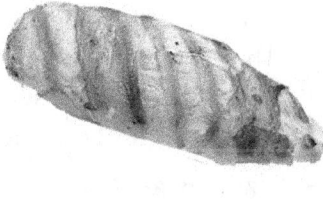

- Lamb
- Turkey
- Organ meat

## Fish & Seafood

Wild caught is better for you than farm raised.

- All fish
- Crab

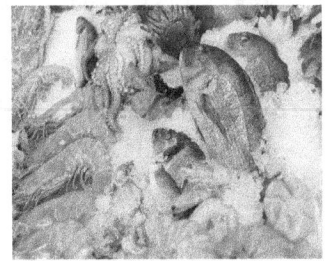

- Shrimp
- Lobster
- Clams

- Oysters
- Mussels

**Fats and Oils**

- Clarified butter
- Ghee
- Coconut oil
- Extra virgin olive oil
- Avocado
- Coconut butter
- Coconut milk
- Olives
- Nut and seed butters, including, peanut, sunflower seed and almond, 100% pure without added sugar.

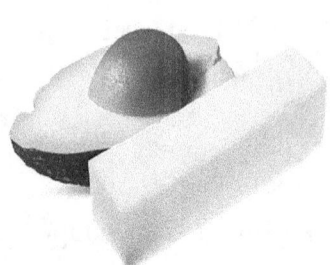

**Beans**

Fresh dried beans are best—they come straight from the plant.

Avoid Canned products if at all possible. Canned goods have the natural enzymes removed. Enzymes are the workers of the body—they make things happen and are involved in many body processes as well as memory function. Check the label and look out for various added ingredients that turn the original whole food into a processed one. Things to look for include, but are not limited to: cane syrup, salt, high fructose corn syrup, calcium chloride (added as a firming agent), disodium EDTA (added to retain color.)

- Adzuki Beans
- Black Beans/Black Turtle Beans
- Black-Eyed Peas
- Butter Beans
- Fava Beans/Broad Beans
- Flageolet Beans
- Garbanzo Beans/Chickpeas
- Kidney Beans

- Lentils—Green, Red, Yellow, Brown, Other
- Lima Beans/Butter Beans
- Navy Beans
- Pigeon Peas
- Pinto Beans
- Red Beans/Small Red Beans
- Scarlet Runner Beans
- Soybeans
- Split Peas—Green, Yellow

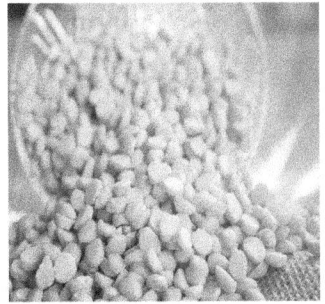

## All Nuts

Eaten raw or roasted and in their natural state without any flavoring or coatings.

- Almonds
- Walnuts
- Macadamia
- Pecans
- Cashew
- Peanuts
- Hazelnuts
- Brazil nuts

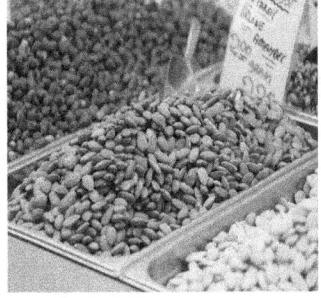

## Seeds

- Pumpkin
- Sunflower
- Chia
- Flax seeds
- Sesame seeds

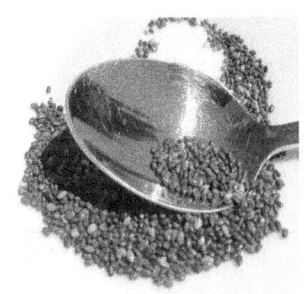

**Herbs & Spices**

Fresh organic or wild crafted herbs are always best.

- Basil
- Cumin seeds
- Garlic
- Dill
- Mint
- Marjoram
- Ginger
- Mustard seeds
- Oregano
- Parsley
- Peppermint
- Rosemary
- Sage
- Thyme
- Turmeric
- Black pepper
- Chili pepper, dried
- Cilantro & Coriander seeds
- Cinnamon, ground
- Cloves

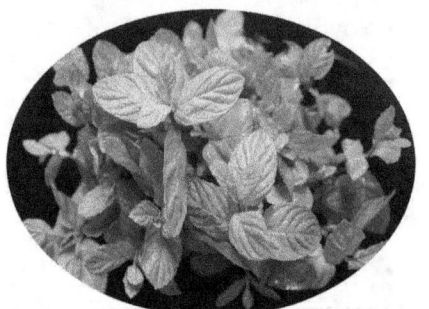

**Beverages**

- Filtered or bottled water (not tap water which in many areas is full of chemicals)
- Milk
- 100% pure fruit juice (not from concentrate), including Aloe Vera juice
- 100% pure vegetable juice (not from concentrate)

- Plain coffee

- Tea—plain with no sugar or flavoring added

- Green tea (fresh brewed at home, or 100% pure, with nothing added, bottled versions)

**Sweeteners and Flavors (in moderation)**

- Raw organic honey

- 100% maple syrup

- Fruit juice concentrates

- Raw cacao nibs

- Raw cocoa powder

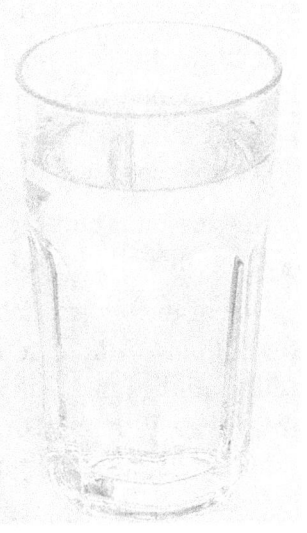

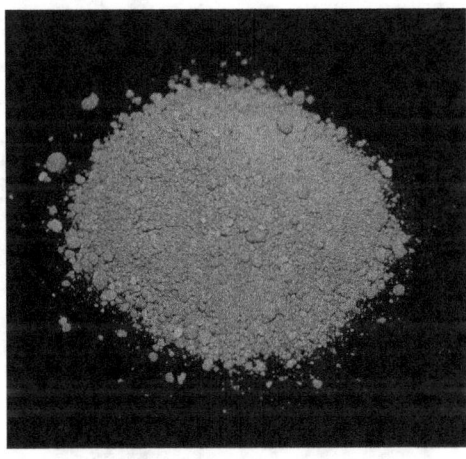

# Chapter 9

## How to Change to a Wholesome Diet

For many individuals changing to a wholesome diet can be a really life changing experience. You have to bear in mind that this is a process—of changing a taste pattern developed over possible a long period of time, to one which will be based on wholesome food that many of our taste buds have forgotten about.

It could possibly take time, and certainly a degree of dedication, but, remember the benefits can be substantial, and certainly as we age, the effects of an unhealthy lifestyles can manifest itself in our 40's and beyond and the consequences can at times be overwhelming.

However, it is never too late to start to make beneficial changes that will significantly improve our health, wellness and wellbeing!

One of the biggest decisions is how and when to start. If you have the willpower and determination you can make the decision to stop eating all the junk food right now and start on a whole food lifestyle immediately, though, this can prove difficult for some. The other option is to start gradually and build up. You know what your capabilities are yourself, so it is you who has to make the decision.

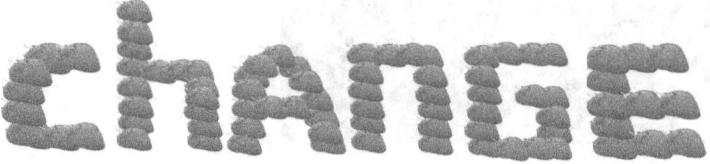

So once you have made the commitment go ahead and do it. As you get used to this new way of eating, it will become easier to follow your new healthy lifestyle each and every day.

For those of you who need more help, here are some suggestions.

### Build Up Gradually

One of the easiest ways to get into wholesome eating is to make small gradual changes rather than try and do it all at once. Consider making food substitutions on a regular basis. By focusing on small achievable results over time, can go a long way to changing habits that have quite possibly been with us since childhood.

This method can prove effective because easing into a new program gradually, can eliminate any signs of frustration or burnout, that can result in some individuals giving up on the new wholesome lifestyle altogether.

## Where Should You Start?

You could start by eliminating one or two unhealthy items from your diet each week. Then keep adding more weekly.

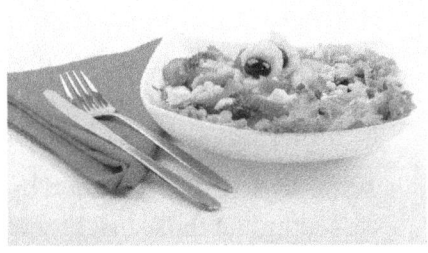

Begin to notice the changes in how you feel, in the weight you start to lose and in new found energy that you have. Then build on that.

Before long you will be living the whole food lifestyle and enjoying all the benefits that eating wholesome foods brings.

## And what About Sodas and Other Unhealthy Drinks?

- Exchange soda for bottled water (ideally plain not sparkling), plain pure green tea or fresh brewed ice tea. Why not consider starting juicing at home, where you can juice vegetables and fruits as healthier options to soda.
- If you typically drink Frappuccino drinks at your favorite coffee house, exchange for plain coffee with a splash of real cream.

## Snack Evaluation

Snacks are typical culprits of processed junk food, so, assess your snack intake and exchange for healthier options.

- If you eat chips, choose plain nuts instead, they will still satisfy your crunch cravings.
- Exchange fruit roll ups and candy for fresh fruit.

## Eliminate the Candy

This one is difficult for most of us because we are addicted to sugary fatty foods, but, it needs to be considered and probably more than anything else.

- Begin in a small way by substitut-
  ing at least 3 pieces of candy each
  week with fruit and keep increasing the numbers of substitutions
  weekly. Bear in mind that fruits
  contain natural sugar, therefore
  they are naturally sweet, and
  they can satisfy that craving for
  something sweet in a much more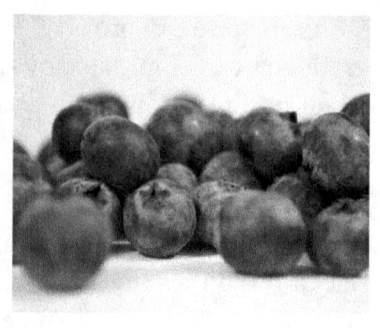
  healthier way than cookies, donuts, Danish and cake.

- 100% cacao nibs are a good option as they are whole, and unprocessed unlike those brightly wrapped candy bars you see stacked
  up at the supermarket checkout line.

**When Eating Out**

Eating out at restaurants and certain fast food joints is often bad
news. When you eat out you have no control over the ingredients that
have gone into your food or how it was prepared. In addition, fast
food places are loaded with processed foods that are not conducive
to wholesome eating.

But, there are smart choices to fast food eating too, so, if you can
stand the temptation and avoid ordering junk, then even McDonalds
has fresh salads. Places like, El Pollo Loco offer fresh grilled chicken
and fresh tomato salsa. Many restaurants offer fresh grilled fish and
chicken and steamed plain vegetables.

In the end, it all really depends on what you order and the questions
you ask.

When you first commence a program of healthy eating, you have to
learn to make the right choices, but, if the burger and fries is calling
your name and too hard to resist then just try and stay away.

**Cooking At Home**

When you prepare and cook food at home you are in control of the
ingredients, and with a whole food lifestyle this is crucial.

# Chapter 10

# And What About Water

As part of your wholefood program, you also have to consider the quality of water you drink as well.

Water is essential for life! And it makes up about 60 per cent of your body weight. You can go for an extended time without food, but water—you will only stay alive for about three days without drinking it. Why is that? Well, water is needed by every system of your body. Water flushes toxins out of vital organs; it also carries nutrients from the food to body cells. In addition, it provides a moist environment for ear, throat and nose tissues.

Each day you lose water through your normal body functions such as breathing, perspiration, urine and bowel movements. In order for your body to function normally, it is important to replenish its water supply by consuming liquids and foods that contain water.

**There are three types of drinking water:**

1. Tap water

2. Bottled water

3. Filtered water.

Tap water is the worst of the three for you to drink. It is contaminated with a host of chemicals that are added by your state or municipal water authority. As an example, I am sure you have heard of fluoride. So where does fluoride come from? It does occur naturally in the environment; however, the fluoride added to the water supply is a hazardous byproduct of the fertilizer industry. This toxic substance has never been required to undergo any clinical trials to determine its safety or effectiveness.

In fact, studies have shown that fluoride has a negative effect on the pineal gland in the brain as well as other neurological processes which may be linked to Alzheimer's disease.

Fluoride is commonly found in toothpaste where we are told that it helps protect teeth against decay. But the US Food and Drug Administration (FDA) classifies fluoride as an "unapproved drug".

What about bottled water? Did you know that 40 per cent of bottled water is actually tap water? Take one well-known brand. It states on the label that it is "purified water". This basically means it is either tap or river water that has been put through a filtration process.

Have you heard (or tried) vitamin water because on the face of it—this seems to be a better choice for your health? Unfortunately, vitamin waters are little more than a clever marketing gimmick and are as unhealthy as drinking sodas. Vitamin water contains excessive levels of high fructose corn syrup, artificial colors, additives preservatives and caffeine. All things I have mentioned in this book you should avoid.

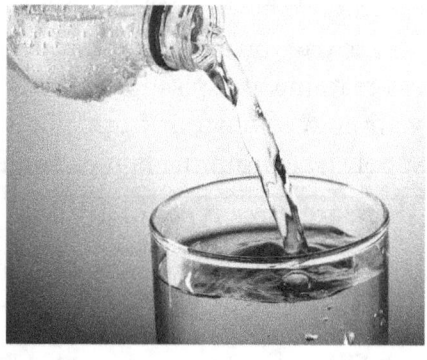

So what is the best type of bottled water? That which comes straight out of the ground which contains natural minerals. Do a little research. Bottled mineral water contains a label with an assay of the mineral content. Some mineral water contains more of certain minerals than others. But they are a better choice than all the clever marketing hype of purified water and vitamin water.

Oh, and one final thing whilst we are on the subject of on bottled water. Avoid plastic bottles if at all possible. Glass bottles are best. Plastic bottles are made from plastic which contains a chemical called bisphenol A or BPA. This is a synthetic hormone disrupter which has been linked to various health problems including:

- Learning and behavioral problems
- Altered immune system function
- Prostate and breast cancer
- Risk of obesity
- Early puberty in both males and females

Not only that, the amount of discarded plastic bottles globally is staggering and causes great harm to the environment.

So which type of water is best?  Well, it comes back to tap water, but this time with a filtration system added. There are various types as follows:

### Reverse Osmosis Filter

An RO filter will remove approximately 80 per cent of the fluoride as well as chlorine, and organic and inorganic contaminants in your water. The downside of installing an RO system is that you will probably need the services of a plumber for the installation; another disadvantage is the cost of the unit.

### Ion Exchange Filter

This type of filter was originally developed for industrial applications before being developed for in home use. It removes dissolved salts such as calcium which occur naturally in the water. The system helps soften the water and as a result, has the effect of reducing scale build-up. The system actually exchanges natural forming mineral ions in the water with its own ions.

### Granular Carbon Filter Units

These are probably the most popular and least expensive types of water filter for use on the counter top or under the counter. Granular carbon filters which need changing as advised by the manufacturer, remove contaminants from the water. The EPA recognizes granular activated carbon filters as being the best available technology for removing organic and industrial chemicals from the water.

### How Much Filtered Water Should You Drink Each Day

It is often suggested that eight glasses of filtered water each day should be the average. But, bear in mind that some people may need to drink more than others. As a good guide, you should drink sufficient filtered water each day to turn the color of your urine a pale yellow.

You may need to increase your water consumption if you are in a hot climate or involved in strenuous activities to prevent dehydration.

Also, as you age your thirst mechanism tends to work less effectively. Therefore close attention should be made to the color of the urine to ensure that adequate amounts of filtered water are consumed each day.

# Chapter 11

# A Day In The Life Of A Whole Food Diet

## Breakfast

Breakfast could take several different forms.

## Quick Breakfast

If you are pushed for time, then consider eating full-fat plain yogurt with fresh fruit. It is important to make sure that the yogurt is plain and contains no added sugar or fats. Try and get organic yogurt if you can.

## Alternative Breakfasts

Try a bowl of steel-cut oats with low-fat milk, plus fresh fruits such as blueberries or raspberries, raw honey and walnuts.

Alternatively, if you have the time, you could prepare a cooked breakfast.

Make an omelet out of cage free organic eggs, whole cheese and vegetables. You can add fresh parmesan or feta cheese and broccoli, mushrooms, onions, tomatoes, spinach or zucchini.

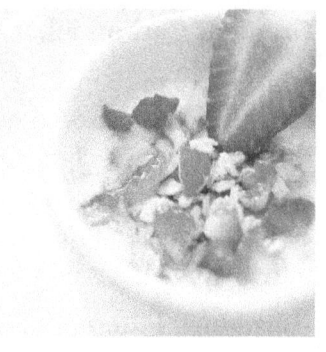

An easier to prepare breakfast could include cage free organic eggs (boiled or poached—not fried)and whole wheat toast with farm raised butter. Another option is a whole grain cereal (check ingredients), Grape Nuts are also a good choice, with whole milk and berries on top.

## Lunch

Be sure to include a protein source, vegetables, and a healthy source of fat in your lunches and dinners.

## Chicken Salad

Consider making a large green salad with fresh lettuce and any of these vegetables: sliced cherry tomatoes, avocado, spring onions, carrots, celery, green beans, water cress and cucumbers.

Season with a hint of olive oil and combine it with an organic, roasted chicken breast. This will make a great whole meal lunch.

If you would like to add more flavor to your meal, you can make a salad dressing with orange juice, olive oil, red wine vinegar and a hint of soy sauce (read the ingredient label and be aware of unnecessary additions.)

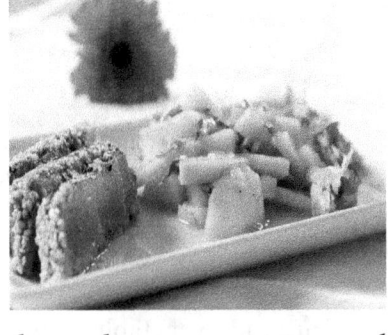

### Grilled Fish

How about making a stir-fry using bean sprouts, carrots, cauliflower and soy sauce (read the label on the soy sauce mentioned above?) You could serve it with a filet of fish, such as tilapia, salmon or tuna on the side.

If you still feel hungry, you can complement either of these lunch dishes with a healthy soup made from broccoli, carrots, potatoes and cilantro.

### Whole Wheat Chicken Pita

Stuff a whole wheat pita with grilled chicken breast, along with fresh raw tomatoes, cucumbers, lettuce, onion, broccoli, spinach, or any vegetables you love. An apple makes for a delicious dessert.

Another option is whole wheat pasta drizzled with extra virgin olive oil tossed with cherry tomatoes, fresh garlic and herbs with shaved parmesan cheese on top. Add grilled shrimp to make it extra hearty.

The many available Quinoa salad recipes make for a great whole lunch as well.

An unprocessed turkey (not lunch meat) sandwich on whole wheat bread with lots of vegetables is another great option for a healthy wholefood lunch.

**Dinner**

Why not try steamed wild salmon with a side of oven-roasted asparagus, seasoned with olive oil, lemon juice and fresh dill or garlic? Add a one cup serving of a whole grain, like brown rice, lentils or a whole wheat roll. If you prefer, you could replace the salmon with tilapia, catfish, scallops, shrimp or chicken.

You can also eat a grilled lean steak with a side of steamed vegetables and quinoa or brown rice. Roasted sweet potatoes and black beans make a great side dish as well.

A grilled turkey breast with a side of mushrooms grilled with fresh butter and garlic and a vegetable/barley pilaf makes for a great dinner.

**Snacks**

- Dairy products, such as, feta cheese, parmesan cheese and plain, natural yogurt can be enjoyed as whole food snacks.

- You could also make your own guacamole or hummus (chickpea spread) and dip carrots, celery or cucumbers.

- Plain boiled eggs

- Nuts

- Fruits and vegetables also make up healthy whole food snacks

- How about fruits and vegetables, like celery and apples with 100% nut butter, such as almond or peanut butter on top.

- Make smoothies out of pureed, fresh fruit, plain yogurt and whole raw milk.

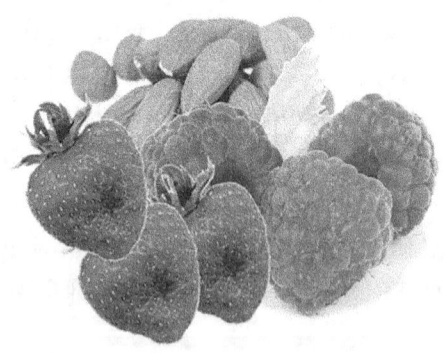

# Chapter 12

## 45 Whole Food Substitutions For Processed Favorites

It is quite possible to substitute certain unhealthy, processed foods with whole foods.

1. Grilled chicken breast rather than chicken nuggets.

2. A baked potato with chopped green onions and sour cream rather than a bag of sour cream and onion potato chips.

3. Fresh strawberries with plain organic yogurt rather than a strawberry sundae.

4. Fresh fruit and plain organic yogurt smoothie rather than an ice cream shake.

5. Thinly sliced home cooked roasts, hams and meats rather than lunch meat and cold cuts that contain nitrates, preservatives and additives to extend shelf life, and high fructose corn syrup.

6. Butter rather than margarine.

7. Whole grain pasta or spaghetti squash rather than white pasta.

8. Brown rice rather than white rice.

9. Celtic or Himalayan sea salt rather than iodized commercial table salt that contains sugar fillers and chemicals.

10. Whole wheat flour, spelt flour or sprouted grain flour rather than white flour that is devoid of any nutrients and made from wheat that has been sprayed heavily with pesticides and insecticides, and in many cases bleach has been added.

11. Apple slices sprinkled with fresh cinnamon rather than cinnamon pop tarts.

12. Raw organic honey rather than white sugar.

13. Whole oranges or 100% pure orange juice rather than orange drinks.

14. Fresh whole strawberries (or any fruit) rather than strawberry Jell-O.

15. Fresh vegetables rather than canned varieties.

16. Fresh whole blueberries with raw (unpasteurized) cream rather than blueberry pop tarts.

17. Dried beans (black, red, kidney, etc.) prepared at home versus canned beans.

18. Fresh whole fruit rather than fruit cups or fruit cocktail products.

19. Fresh figs rather than fig sandwich cookies.

20. 70% cocoa dark chocolate with no sugar added. 100% pure peanut or almond butter rather than peanut butter cup candy.

21. Fresh corn rather than corn chips or corn flakes.

22. Fresh spinach rather than frozen creamed spinach products.

23. Fresh whole garlic rather than ready-made jarred minced garlic or bottled garlic marinades.

24. Fresh homemade soups rather than canned varieties.

25. Grass fed beef rather than grain/corn fed beef.

26. Cage free raised eggs rather than egg beaters or caged chicken eggs.

27. Fresh raw cream rather than flavored coffee creamers and fat free half and half.

28. Plain low-fat or nonfat yogurt rather than flavored yogurts and yogurt drinks.

29. Whole peanuts and 100% nothing added peanut butter rather than peanut butter products.

30. Whole Edamame rather than store bought soy burgers.

31. Tomatoes crushed/pureed at home rather than ketchup.

32. Steel-cut oatmeal rather than instant oatmeal products.

33. Thinly sliced and crisped in oven potato slices rather than potato chips.

34. Homemade ice cream with raw cream and fresh fruit rather than store bought ice cream.

35. Whole wheat crust pizza with grass fed raw milk mozzarella cheese, fresh crushed tomato sauce and fresh vegetables rather than "regular" pizza.

36. Baked sweet potato slices rather than French fries.

37. Fruit flavored seltzer water or plain seltzer with fresh lime or lemon rather than soda.

38. Baked whole apple with raisins and cinnamon rather than apple pie.

39. Grass fed beef or turkey burger with raw vegetables wrapped in lettuce or on a whole wheat bun rather than a regular burger.

40. Raisins or dried fruit rather than candy.

41. Organic stove popped popcorn that contains no added chemicals or preservatives rather than bagged microwave popcorn products.

42. Organic probiotic plain yogurt with fresh berries rather than ice-cream.

43. Homemade crushed ice and fresh fruit smoothies rather than popsicles.

44. Onions grilled in canola or coconut oil rather than onion rings.

45. Make buckwheat pancakes rather than white flour pancakes.

# Chapter 13

## 36 Whole Food Cooking And Eating Tips

Wholesome eating is really simple once you understand food and its origins. Where did it come from? Has it been processed and unhealthy ingredients added? Rather than focusing on managing food choices, simply, cook and eat more natural foods rather than their processed counterparts, and always be mindful of the pathway between a food's origins and your plate.

So how do you go about getting more whole foods into your diet? It's not as hard as you may think.

Here are 36 tips:

1. Homemade is the best way to ensure you get a healthy whole food diet. Ready-made products are convenient, but, they always contain additives, preservatives, sugar, added salt and other unnecessary ingredients. Many packaged foods are not "real" food at all.

2. Whole food cooking takes more preparation time than buying ready-made processed products, so, prepare and plan ahead for the week and have everything ready in advance. For example, you can chop up vegetables, put them into freezer bags, and freeze to use throughout the week.

3. Farmer's markets are the best places to find locally grown organic fruits and vegetables, along with organic meats, fresh nuts and even natural dairy products.

4. When cooking whole food, the goal is to maintain its natural integrity as much as possible. For example, grilling chicken breasts in their natural state without coating them in bread crumbs.

5. Steaming and poaching are some of the best options for whole food cooking. This especially applies to fish, poultry and vegetables in terms of preserving nutritional value and keeping the food's natural integrity.

6. Freezing is a great way to have ready made on hand whole food meals available for busy work days.

7. Prepare and cook a variety of foods to get the most nutritional value.

8. If you really dislike eating whole vegetables, juice them instead and add sweetness with low sugar fruits, like lemons, limes, apples and even ginger.

9. Buy fruits and vegetables when in season to save money.

10. Eat food in its raw state as much as possible, this means fresh fruits, vegetables and nuts.

11. Traditional breakfast foods are loaded with processed items. As an alternative, make fresh vegetable omelets with organic cage free eggs, nonfat yogurt with fresh fruit, and steel-cut oatmeal with fresh fruit. Substitute hash browns with roasted sweet potatoes.

12. Choose a rainbow of colors in vegetables, this ensures you get a good supply of nutrients and antioxidants.

13. Only shop around the inside edge of the supermarket food department, this is where all the whole foods are to be found. All the inside aisles house mostly processed foods.

14. Prepare fresh vegetables at the weekend and save them in well-sealed freezer bags for use during busy work days.

15. Almond flour is a great substitute for unhealthy white flour in muffins. Search online for recipes—there are loads of them!

16. The crockpot is a whole food eater's best friend. Simply add in fresh herbs, vegetables, an organic beef round, turkey legs or a whole organic chicken on top. Then add some water, fresh tomatoes and garlic cloves. Turn it on before you leave for work and get home to a fine meal. There are literally hundreds of crockpot whole food dishes ready and waiting to be savored. You can prepare all the ingredients for individual recipes and place them into freezer bags to have on hand for the week. Look online for recipe ideas.

17. Replace white flour with whole-wheat flour.

18. Use whole wheat pasta, brown rice and quinoa in all your recipes and for side dishes.

19. Make whole wheat crust for homemade pizza.

20. Steam fresh vegetables rather than using canned products.

21. Use butter for cooking rather than processed products like lard and margarine.

22. Make homemade soups with all natural ingredients rather than using canned varieties. Soup can be made in bulk and frozen for fast access to wholesome goodness.

23. Use a food processor to make your own ketchup with fresh tomatoes and without added sugar and preservatives.

24. Store purchased ready-made side dishes, like pasta, rice and potato products are all processed and loaded with additives, preservatives and other unwanted ingredients. Make homemade instead: potatoes au gratin, rice with broccoli and cheese and pastas can all be made at home with whole ingredients and without additives.

25. Buy fresh chicken, turkey and beef rather than ready-made products, like, chicken nuggets and beef patties.

26. Crush fresh berries and spread onto whole wheat toast rather than using preserves.

27. Make fresh marinara sauce at home rather than buying canned or bottled products that have preservatives, too much sodium, sugar and other unnecessary ingredients added.

28. Make healthy cookies with steel-cut oats, raisins and stevia rather than refined sugar.

29. Grill chicken and fish without adding a coating or bread crumbs. Fish sticks and chicken nuggets are processed foods.

30. Make homemade ice cream using raw cream and fresh fruits rather than buying processed ice cream products that are often loaded with extra ingredients.

31. Blend fresh fruit and organic yogurt in a blender to make healthier shake varieties.

32. Popsicles are loaded with sugar, instead, blend fresh fruit in a blender and freeze in Popsicle ice trays to make healthy fruit pops for kids.

33. It is easy to make your own peanut butter without additives or added sugar. Chop up 2 cups of raw or roasted peanuts in a

food processor, then slowly blend in 1½ teaspoons of vegetable or canola oil until you get the consistency you desire, either smooth or chunky.

34. Use fresh herbs like garlic, basil and parsley in all your recipes to add flavor.

35. Store purchased juice drinks are full of sugar and little nutrition. Make your own juice drinks at home using vegetables and low sugar fruits, like granny smith apples, lemons, limes and grapefruits.

36. Homemade bread is a wonderful way to ensure that only natural ingredients go in and baking your own allows you to use the best whole wheat flours. Buying a good quality bread making machine is a sound investment, as it reduces the kneading time considerably. Most bread machines come with a recipe book containing some amazing bread recipes.

# Chapter 14

## 3 High Fiber Whole Food Recipes

**Baked Chickpeas**

Serves: 2

Ingredients

- 1 (14 1/2oz) can chickpeas, (rinsed and drained)
- 4 tbsp. fresh parsley (chopped)
- 1 tsp. ground cumin
- 3 cloves garlic (minced)
- 1/4 tsp. ground coriander
- 1/4 tsp. baking soda
- 1/4 tsp. salt
- 4 tbsp. onion (chopped) (pressed)
- 1 tbsp. plain flour
- 1 egg (beaten)
- 2 tsp. olive oil

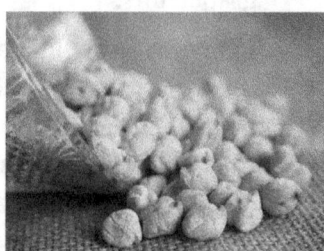

Instructions

1. Preheat oven to 390 F.
2. Into a food processor, combine chickpeas, cumin, coriander, parsley, garlic, baking soda and salt. Process until pureed.
3. Transfer mixture into a bowl; add pressed onions and mix to blend.
4. Mix in flour and egg, mix until well incorporated.
5. Form patties, 3 inch in diameter. Set aside for 12 minutes
6. Heat oil over a medium flame in a large, oven-safe frying pan.
7. Fry patties for about 3 minutes per side or until golden brown. Transfer into oven and heat for about 10 minutes.
8. Serve with whole wheat pita bread.

## Mixed Vegetables And Quinoa Stuffed Peppers

Makes 6 servings

Ingredients

- 1 cup Quinoa
- 2 cups vegetable stock
- 6 red and green bell peppers, (halved and seeded)
- 4 tbsp. coconut oil
- Salt and freshly ground black pepper (to taste)
- 4 cloves garlic (thinly sliced)
- 1 small to medium firm zucchini (seeded and chopped)

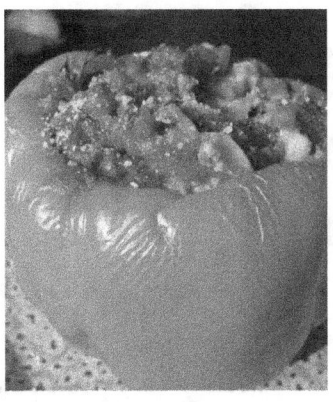

- 1 small firm eggplant (trimmed, chopped)
- 1 red onion (chopped)
- 1 fresh chili pepper (thinly sliced)
- 2 plum tomatoes (chopped)
- 1/2 cup fresh flat-leaf parsley leaves (chopped)
- 1/4 cup fresh mint leaves (chopped)
- 2 tbsp. olive oil
- 1 cup feta cheese (crumbled for topping)

Instructions

1. Preheat oven to 450 F.
2. Prepare Quinoa in a pot with vegetable stock (or chicken stock) for about 15 minutes or until it's tender and fluffy.
3. Lower oven temperature to 374 F.
4. Brush bell peppers with oil and season with salt and pepper. Place on a baking tray, uncut sides up and roast for about 20 minutes or until tender and skins start to darken.
5. Cool on wire rack.

6. Meantime, heat 3 tbsp. oil in a saucepan over a medium-heat. Sauté garlic for about 30 seconds or until browned. Mix in onions, zucchini, eggplant, and chili peppers. Cook for about 10 minutes or until tender.

7. Add cooked quinoa, and the rest of the ingredients.

8. Season with salt and pepper.

9. Stuff peppers with the mixture, drizzle with olive oil and heat inside oven for several minutes until heated through.

10. Top with cheese and serve.

## Zucchini & Turkey Pasta

Ingredients

- 2 large zucchinis (shredded into spirals, use a food processor or a handy gadget, like the SpiraLife Vegetable Spiralizer that turns zucchini into pasta shaped spirals)
- 2 tbsp. of extra virgin olive oil
- 1/2 medium red onion (chopped)
- 1/2 celery stalk (diced)
- 1/2 carrot (diced)

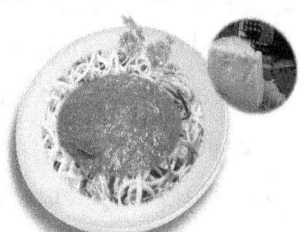

- 1 tsp. of red hot pepper flakes
- 2 medium cloves of garlic (minced)
- 2 cups of fresh crushed tomatoes
- 3/4 tbsp. of tomato paste
- Salt and pepper to taste
- 1/4 cup of organic chicken broth
- 1/3 cup of fresh basil (chopped)
- 1 tbsp. of fresh or flaked oregano
- 1/2 lb. of ground turkey
- Fresh whole shredded parmesan cheese (don't use prepared products)

Instructions

1. Into a food processor, combine carrots and celery; pulse until almost pureed with some chunky bits remaining, put aside.

2. Into a large pan, heat oil over medium heat; season with salt and pepper and sauté garlic for about 30 seconds or until browned.

3. Mix in pepper flakes, sauté for 30 seconds then stir in onions. Sauté for another 2 min. or until translucent.

4. Combine in blended carrot-celery mixture and cook for about 1 minute.

5. Set vegetables on the sides of the pan and put turkey in the center of the pan. Cook by loosening the chunks, add a pinch of oregano flakes and cook further until light brown.

6. Mix the vegetables with the turkey, add a little more oregano flakes, pour in broth and continue cooking until most of the water evaporates.

7. Put in tomatoes, tomato paste and remaining oregano flakes. Bring to the boil and simmer over lower heat for about 15 min. or until sauce is reduced.

8. Season with salt and pepper, and then add the basil leaves.

9. Mix in the zucchini pasta and stir thoroughly to combine.

10. Plate and garnish with Parmesan cheese before serving.

# Part Two
## The Need For Dietary Supplements
### Why Vitamins, Minerals, Essential Fatty Acids And Enzymes Are So Important

# Chapter 15

# Supplements, Free Radicals and Antioxidants

At the beginning of this book I discussed a "balanced diet" and "we get everything from our food", as I explained that is not the case. Listening to the so called "experts", they never actually say what a balanced diet is. It is just a sweeping statement that encompasses everyone and everything, when in fact no two people are exactly alike. Everyone has different dietary needs as well as different lifestyles.

In his book *Biochemical Individuality* Dr Roger Williams, who discovered vitamin B5 (pantothenic acid), explains how each person has organs that are different shapes and sizes, how each person has different levels of enzymes and different requirements for vitamins and minerals. A ten fold difference in requirements from one person to another is not unusual. So how come we get everything we need from a balanced diet, without saying what a balanced diet is.

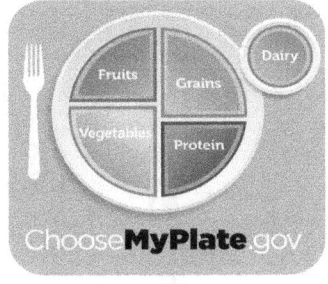

The only light that is shed on the 'balanced diet" is to refer to the basic food groups: grains, dairy products, meat, fish and poultry, fruits and vegetables which the United States Department of Agriculture (USDA) promotes through its 'Choose My Plate" program. However, if you listen to a recording of *Dead Doctors Don't Lie* by Dr Joel Wallach, he explains how he conducted hundreds of autopsies which revealed that the vast majority of deaths were caused by diseases brought on by nutritional deficiencies.

People tend to eat for taste, not nutrition, and it can be very difficult to change a person's eating habits. It is a fact that junk food tastes good and people will not be told to eat fruit and vegetables. This is one reason why informed people understand the importance of supplementing the modern diet with extra vitamins, minerals, antioxidants and other nutrients. The old adage that we get everything from our diet and that supplementing with vitamins and minerals is just creating expensive urine has been knocked on the head. It is well researched that we no longer get everything we need nutritionally from our diet.

People who say that they are well off and eat a good diet, therefore they don't need supplements, don't always understand why they need antioxidants. Antioxidants scavenge free radicals a major source of which is the highly processed food of an affluent society.

Finally, if you do a vigorous exercise regime or play sports where a lot of activity is involved, then your body will generate further free radicals. In order to protect your cells, joints and tissues, it is advisable to increase your intake of antioxidants to counteract this extra free radical activity.

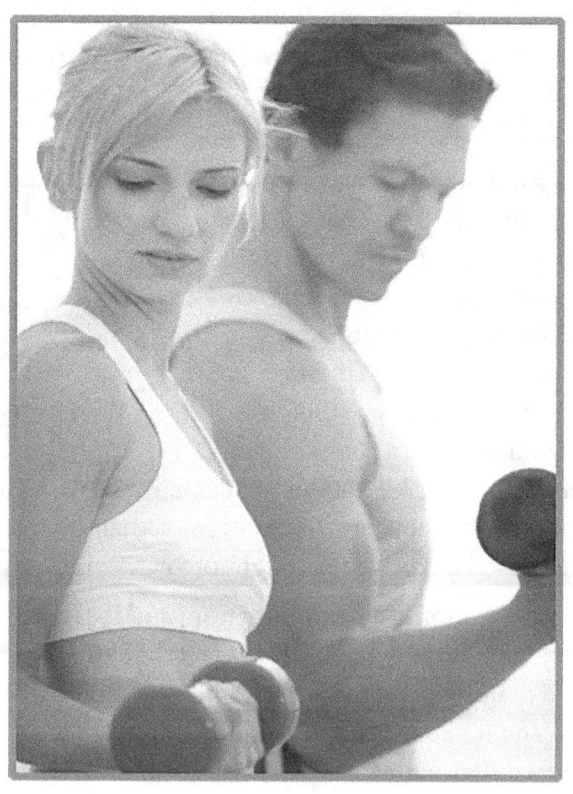

# Chapter 16

# Understanding Free Radicals and Antioxidants

What are free radicals? Why do they damage the human body? How is it that vitamin A, E and C as well as beta carotene help protect the body from free radical damage? It is important to understand why eating at least five serving each day of antioxidant rich fruits and vegetables along with suitable antioxidant supplements will benefit your health, and help prevent cancer, heart disease and other illnesses from developing.

To start, let us look at free radicals. Where do they come from, and what damage do they do. Everyone has free radicals—they are part of living. They come from the metabolism of the food you eat as well as from environmental factors such as air pollution, radiation, cigarette smoke, herbicides, household cleaners, skin care products, cosmetics—in fact anything that has a chemical element in it. Even the immune system can develop free radicals to help destroy bacteria and viruses.

Free radicals are atoms or groups of atoms with an odd or un-paired number of electrons. These can be formed when oxygen interacts with certain molecules.

These highly reactive molecules can start a chain reaction—like a falling pack of cards. The danger is the damage they can do when they come into contact with important cellular components such as DNA or cell membranes. Cells can die if this occurs.

Some of the degenerative conditions caused by free radicals include:

- Deterioration of the eye lens, which contributes to cataracts or blindness.
- Inflammation of the joints (arthritis).
- Damage to nerve cells in the brain, which can result in Parkinson's or Alzheimer's disease.
- Acceleration of the aging process.
- Increased risk of coronary heart disease since free radicals encourage low-density lipoprotein (LDL) cholesterol to adhere to artery walls in the form of arterial plaque.
- Certain cancers triggered by damaged cell DNA.

This is where antioxidants come in. The main antioxidant vitamins are vitamin A, beta carotene, vitamin C and vitamin E. There are also antioxidant minerals such as selenium and zinc, and antioxidant herbs such as ginkgo biloba and garlic which support the circulatory system.

Antioxidants neutralize free radicals by donating one of their own electrons thus ending the electron stealing cycle. The antioxidants don't become free radicals themselves as they have spare electrons and are stable in either form. They act as protectors and help to prevent tissue and cell damage which could lead to various diseases.

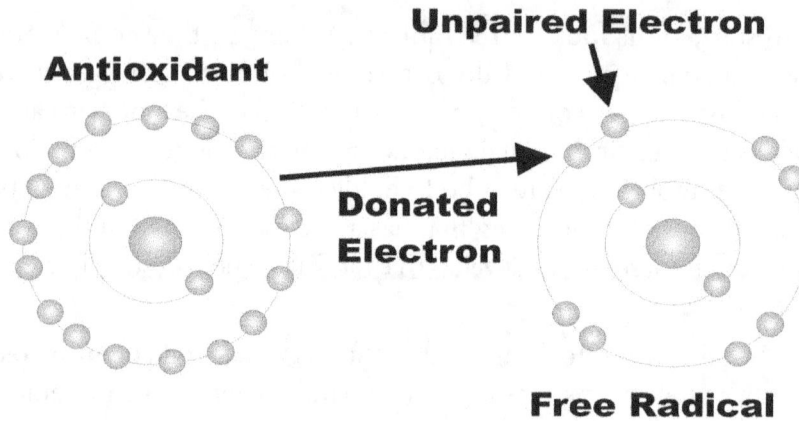

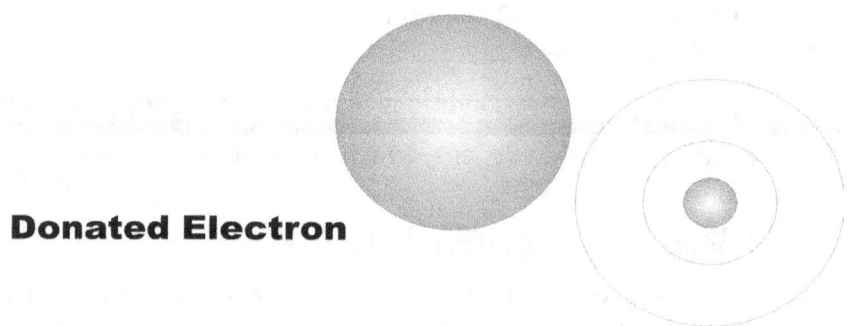

# Chapter 17

## Antioxidants and Disease Prevention

The greatest killers in the Western world are heart disease, stroke and cancer. Vitamin E is the most abundant fat soluble antioxidant in the body. It is one of the main defenders against oxidation and helps protect you against cardiovascular disease by helping to neutralize the effects of LDL (low density lipoprotein)—the "bad" cholesterol and plaque formation which blocks arteries and can lead to a heart attack or stroke.

The most abundant water soluble antioxidant is vitamin C. Vitamin C helps to neutralize free radical formations caused by cigarette smoke and other forms of air pollution. Also many studies have shown that high doses of vitamin C equate to lower rates of cancer especially of the mouth, larynx and esophagus.

So, along with your five servings each day of antioxidant rich fruit and vegetables, you may want to consider topping up with extra antioxidant supplements: vitamin E, C and beta carotene as well.

Some good sources of antioxidants include:

- **Allium sulfur compounds**—leeks, onions and garlic
- **Anthocyanins**—eggplant, grapes and berries
- **Beta-carotene**—pumpkin, mangoes, apricots, carrots, spinach and parsley
- **Catechins**—red wine and green tea
- **Copper**—seafood, lean meat, milk and nuts
- **Cryptoxanthins**—red capsicum, pumpkin and mangoes
- **Flavonoids**—tea, green tea, citrus fruits, red wine, onions and apples
- **Indoles**—cruciferous vegetables such as broccoli, cabbage and cauliflower
- **Isoflavonoids**—soybeans, tofu, lentils, peas and milk
- **Lignans**—sesame seeds, bran, whole grains and vegetables
- **Lutein**—leafy greens like spinach and corn

- **Lycopene**—tomatoes, pink grapefruit and watermelon
- **Manganese**—seafood, lean meat, milk and nuts
- **Polyphenols**—thyme and oregano
- **Selenium**—seafood, offal, lean meat and whole grains
- **Vitamin C**—oranges, blackcurrants, kiwi fruit, mangoes, broccoli, spinach, capsicum and strawberries
- **Vitamin E**—vegetable oils (such as wheat germ oil), avocados, nuts, seeds and whole grains
- **Zinc**—seafood, lean meat, milk and nuts
- **Zoochemicals**—red meat, offal, and fish. (Also derived from the plants that animals eat)

# Chapter 18

# The Need for Supplements

So let us now have a look at supplements and see where they fit in. The subject is so diverse as well as interesting.

One thing to understand is that all supplements are not created equal. There is a vast range available from health food stores, supermarkets, pharmacies and on the Internet. The base material differs also. Some are manufactured from chemical by-products (synthetic) while others are manufactured from natural ingredients.

You have to ask yourself this question. Do you think that something that is manufactured from chemical by-products in a laboratory will have as beneficial an effect in the body as something that is derived from a natural vegetable (or animal) source?

Various tests have been done on synthetic vitamin products and others have been done on natural ones. The natural ones have an "energy factor" which is not available in synthetic ones. Basically natural supplements are a living thing, while something that is synthetic is not.

Even amongst the natural ones, there are differences. It is all to do with the base material. Is it organic or wild crafted (obtained from the wild), or is it from sources that have been treated with chemical fertilizers and pesticides.

It has long been established that you do not get all your daily requirements of vitamins and minerals from the food you eat. This is due to the way crops are grown, the way they are processed and finally how the food that is derived from those crops is prepared in the home. In addition to that, intensive farming methods over the years have depleted the minerals in the soil to such an extent that hardly any exist anymore.

You can refer to the table in chapter 1 to see how much mineral loss takes place in food processing and flour refining.

# Chapter 19

## The RDAs

What are RDAs and what do they do? RDA stands for Recommended Dietary Allowance. They are the RDAs of various vitamins and minerals which are set by governments to prevent such diseases as scurvy; they are not designed to ensure good health.

If you look at the RDAs for various countries, you will see that the recommendations vary wildly. And that is not all. The RDAs do not take into account personal factors such as whether a person smokes, drinks alcohol, lives in a polluted environment, is on the pill, or premenstrual, does a lot of exercise or is under a lot of stress.

Tests have been done by researchers on many adults and the result has been that a high percentage of the participants were lacking in the B vitamins.

As an example, the RDA for vitamin C is set at 80mg for the UK and 90mg for the USA. Yet participants in a research project who took over 400mg of vitamin C per day had fewer incidences of colds. This level of vitamin C is way above the RDA for this vitamin.

Not all nutrients have an RDA. Those that do are on the following table, as well as some of those that don't. The table shows the RDA for the United Kingdom (UK) and the United States (USA). By reviewing the table you will see how the recommendations vary.

| Nutrient | RDA UK | RDA USA |
| --- | --- | --- |
| Vitamin A (mcg) | 800 | 900 |
| Vitamin B1 (mg) | 1.1 | 1.2 |
| Vitamin B2 (mg) | 1.4 | 1.3 |
| Vitamin B3 (mg) | 16 | 16 |
| Vitamin B5 (mg) | 6 | 5 |
| Vitamin B6 (mg) | 1.4 | 1.3 |
| Vitamin B7 (mcg) | 50 | 30 |
| Vitamin B9 (mcg) | 200 | 400 |
| Vitamin B12 (mcg) | 2.5 | 2.4 |
| Vitamin C (mg) | 80 | 90 |
| Vitamin D (mcg) | 5 | 15 |

| Nutrient | RDA UK | RDA USA |
|---|---|---|
| Vitamin E (mg) | 12 | 15 |
| Vitamin K (mcg) | 75 | 12 |
| Biotin (mcg) | 50 | 30 |
| Potassium (mg) | 2000 | 4700 |
| Chloride (mg) | 800 | 2300 |
| Choline (mg) | * | 550 |
| Omega 3 EPA | * | * |
| Omega 6 GLA | * | * |
| Calcium (mg) | 800 | 1000 |
| Chromium (mcg) | 40 | 35 |
| Iodine (mcg) | 150 | 150 |
| Iron (mg) | 14 | 8 |
| Magnesium (mg) | 375 | 400 |
| Manganese (mg) | 2 | 2.3 |
| Selenium (mcg) | 55 | 55 |
| Zinc (mg) | 10 | 11 |
| Phosphorus ((mg) | 700 | 700 |
| Copper (mg) | 1 | 900 (mcg) |
| Flouride (mg) | 3.5 | 10 |
| Molybdenum (mcg) | 50 | 45 |
| Sodium (mg) | 800 | 1500 |

* = No RDA

# Chapter 20

## A Basic Supplement

Selecting a supplement is difficult when you don't have a guide. After all, everyone who sells them says theirs is the best. That's why I worked out the following table to explain what a basic supplement should contain. The best supplement will have all the recognized vitamins and all the minerals except calcium and magnesium at 50 percent of the RDA. It will have some calcium and magnesium, but not 50 percent of the RDA; possibly only 15 percent. The reason is simple: you need so much of these two minerals that they simply won't fit in a pill that contains everything else.

Take a look at the table on the next page. The middle column shows the amount of the nutrient you should get in a supplement. The end columns show it as a percentage of the UK and the USA RDA for average adults.

If you search the pharmacy and health food stores for exactly the same supplement shown in this table, you probably won't find one. Don't despair; simply come as close as possible to it. You might find all the vitamins and minerals, except calcium and magnesium. Take calcium and magnesium as a separate supplement.

The supplement should contain the nutrients shown in the table, in approximately the same ratios to one another; that is the most important criteria—that it is balanced.

Selecting a calcium and mineral supplement depends on the number of dairy products you use and how much your basic supplement contains. If you don't take milk, yogurt or cheese make up for it with a supplement that supplies at least 600mg of calcium and 200mg of magnesium daily. These two essential minerals should not be overlooked.

Is more better? More of some nutrients can help. Compare your body maintenance with that of your car. Keep your car well tuned and serviced and it will respond well to good fuel. Neglect it and you may as well use the cheapest fuel available. If you follow the use of the sensible supplements outlined, you will do just fine. If you feel better using more of some nutrients, it is okay; after all, you are a unique individual and have your own needs.

To sum it all up, natural foods are balanced in fat, protein and carbohydrates and the minerals potassium and sodium. If you eat a wide variety, you will get all your vitamins, minerals and fiber along with your supplement regime. It is important too, that you know what foods cause stress on your body due to a vitamin/mineral imbalance, so that you can avoid them.

| An Excellent Supplement | | | |
|---|---|---|---|
| Nutrient: Vitamins/ Minerals | Supplement Amount | % of UK RDA | % of USA RDA |
| Vitamin A *RE | 500mcg | 63 | 56 |
| Vitamin D | 5mcg | 100 | 33 |
| Vitamin E | 5mg | 42 | 33 |
| Vitamin C | 30mg | 38 | 33 |
| Vitamin B1 | 0.8mg | 73 | 66 |
| Vitamin B2 | 0.8mg | 57 | 62 |
| Vitamin B3 | 10mg | 63 | 62 |
| Vitamin B6 | 1.4mg | 100 | 108 |
| Vitamin 9 | 150mcg | 75 | 38 |
| Vitamin B12 | 1.0mcg | 40 | 42 |
| Calcium | 400mg | 50 | 40 |
| Magnesium | 200mg | 50 | 50 |
| Iron | 6mg | 43 | 75 |
| Zinc | 8mg | 80 | 73 |
| Iodine | 75mcg | 50 | 50 |
| *RE = Retinol Equivalent | | | |

# Chapter 21

## Vitamins for Vitality

So what exactly are vitamins? They each play their own part. They turn on enzymes which are the "spark plugs" that make body functions operate effectively. Vitamins A, C and E are antioxidants which help to neutralize the effects of free radicals in the body. For example, vitamin A from carrots is important for vision and is important for cancer prevention. The B vitamins found in green leafy vegetables help in protein utilization and energy. Vitamin C from such things as oranges helps our bodies to heal when we get a cut, as a protector against the common cold, and as a strengthener of bones and teeth. And vitamin D in milk helps strengthen our bones. We'll have a look in more detail at some of these later.

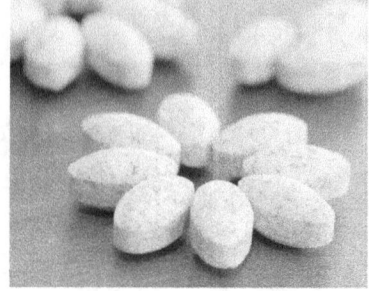

There are two basic types of vitamin:

**Fat soluble.** These are stored in the body's fatty tissue and the liver. They reside in your body until they're needed—some for a few days and some for up to six months. Then special carriers take them to wherever they are needed. Vitamins A, D, E and K are all fat soluble.

**Water soluble.** These are different. When they are water-based they don't tend to get stored in your body as much but travel around in the blood stream. If they are not needed, then, they are expelled in the urine. That means they need to be replaced frequently. These vitamins include vitamin C and the big group of B vitamins—B1 (thiamine), B2 (riboflavin), B3 (niacin), B5 (pantothenic acid), B6 (pyridoxine), B7 (biotin), B9 (folic acid) and B12 (cyanocobalamin), B vitamins are especially important because they not only produce energy but also red blood cells which carry oxygen around your body.

We'll now have a look at each of the vitamins to see exactly why they're important, where they're to be found and the quantities you need to take to preserve your health. I have included the various food sources where each vitamin and mineral is found. However, you can always take a vitamin and / or mineral supplement to rectify any dietary shortfall if required.

**Vitamin A**

Comes in two forms: the animal form called retinol is found in meat, fish, eggs and dairy products, and its precursor—beta carotene which is found in yellow, red, and orange fruit and vegetables. While high levels of vitamin A can be toxic, this is not the case with beta carotene, which the body converts to vitamin A as it is needed. The residue passes out of the body in the urine. Vitamin A is important in maintaining the health of your skin and mucus membranes in places like the nose. It helps strengthen your immune system to help you recover from infections and assists your night vision.

It's found in foods like liver, oily fish such as mackerel, eggs, fortified milk, margarine, butter, cheese, yogurt, carrots, spinach, broccoli, squash, kale and sweet potatoes.

The (RDA): 900mcg (USA) 800mcg (UK).

**Vitamin B1 (Thiamine)**

Thiamine works with other B vitamins to break down food. It also keeps our nerves and muscles in good shape. It is important for maintaining energy levels, for brain function and for good digestion. In addition it assists the body to utilize protein.

We find it in pork, vegetables, milk, cheese, peas, fresh and dried fruit, eggs, wholegrain breads and some breakfast cereals.

The (RDA): 1.2mg (USA) 1.1mg (UK).

**Vitamin B2 (Riboflavin)**

Riboflavin helps maintain the skin, mucous membranes, eyes and the nervous system. It assists in producing steroids and red blood cells and helps the body to absorb iron from food.

You find it in many foods including milk, eggs, breakfast cereals, mushrooms and rice. Riboflavin can be destroyed by ultra violet light so these foods should be kept out of direct sunlight.

The (RDA): 1.3mg (USA) 1.4mg (UK).

**Vitamin B3 (Niacin)**

Niacin like other vitamins helps convert proteins, fats and carbohydrates into energy as well as keeping the digestive and nervous system healthy. It also helps in balancing blood sugar as well as lowering cholesterol levels. There are two types—nicotinic acid and nicotinamide. Like all the B vitamins, they are water soluble so you need them every day.

You get niacin in beef, pork, chicken, wheat flour, maize flour, milk and eggs.

The (RDA): 16mg (USA) 16mg (UK).

### Vitamin B5 (Pantothenic Acid)

Pantothenic acid also helps release the energy from food. It is also used by the adrenal glands to produce stress hormones during periods of physical and psychological stress.

You find it in most meat and vegetables especially chicken, beef, potatoes, porridge oats, tomatoes, kidney, eggs, broccoli, whole grains and rice. Some breakfast cereals are fortified with it.

The (RDA): 5mg (USA) 6mg (UK).

### Vitamin B6 (Pyridoxine)

Pyridoxine is necessary for metabolizing the amino acids in proteins, the formation of antibodies and red blood cells, and for maintaining a healthy digestive and nervous system.

You find B6 in pork, turkey, chicken, bread, cod and whole cereals such as wheat germ, oatmeal and rice. It's also contained in milk, vegetables, eggs, soy milk, peanuts, potatoes and some breakfast cereals.

The (RDA): 1.3mg (USA) 1.4mg (UK).

### Vitamin B7 (Biotin)

Biotin is very important in childhood. It helps your body utilize essential fats and is also important for healthy hair, skin and nails. It also helps turn food into energy as well as being involved in amino acid metabolism. Since its water soluble you need it in your daily diet because it can't be stored.

It's found in a great many foods including kidney, egg yolk and some fruits and vegetables, whole grains, and dried mixed fruit.

The (RDA): 30mcg (USA) 50mcg (UK).

**Vitamin B9 (Folic acid)**

Known as folate in its natural form, it works with B12 to form healthy blood cells and helps reduce the risk of defects in babies such as spina bifida.

Folate is found in small amounts in numerous foods but rich sources are breakfast cereals, some types of bread and fruits such as oranges and bananas. It's also found in broccoli, Brussels sprouts, asparagus, peas, rice and chickpeas.

The (RDA): 400mcg (USA) 200mcg (UK).

**Vitamin B12 (Cyanocobalamin)**

Vitamin B12 helps make red blood cells and generally keeps the nervous system in optimum condition. It helps release energy from the food we eat and it also helps process B9 (folic acid). It deals with the effects of tobacco smoke as well as other toxins in the body. If you don't get enough, you'll probably find that you're anemic. A long term deficiency of B12 can lead to damage of the nervous system. As we get older it becomes more difficult for us to absorb B12.

It's found in fish, meat, poultry and dairy foods. Since you don't get it in vegetables, fruit or grains. Vegans or vegetarians may find themselves deficient in it.

The (RDA): 2.4mcg (USA) 2.5mcg (UK).

Note. All the B vitamins work together. If you are taking vitamin B supplements, it is best to take a Balanced B Complex supplement, that way you can be sure that you are getting your B vitamins in the correct ratios.

If you need more of a particular B vitamin, then you can take this in addition to the Balanced B Complex supplement. As always, make sure that whatever supplement you take it is from a natural source—not synthetic.

**Vitamin C**

This is the one everyone has heard about. It helps protect your body cells and keeps them healthy as well as helping absorb iron from food. It is also used by the adrenal glands to produce hormones and helps to maintain healthy teeth and gums, cartilage, blood vessels and bones.

It is found in fruits such as oranges and kiwi fruit, peppers, broccoli, Brussels sprouts and sweet potatoes.

Compared to other vitamins we need quite a lot every day—minimum 60 mg. However, higher doses are beneficial—up to 2000 mg. It may cause a loose bowel if taken excessively, but this will cease if the dose is reduced. Note! This is not a toxic condition.

The (RDA): 90mg (USA) 80mg (UK).

## Vitamin D

Vitamin D helps regulate the amounts of calcium and phosphorous in the body. These substances keep your teeth and bones healthy.

It's only found in a small number of foods such as liver, oily fish and egg yolk. Other sources include margarine, cheese, butter, breakfast cereals and fortified milk. Most of the vitamin D we get is made in the skin because of its reaction to sunlight. Incidentally, most people—and especially children—lack vitamin D either through a lack of sun exposure, or it is lacking in the diet.

In children, vitamin D is important for proper growth and development. It is also important for the synthesis of calcium. If you're pregnant or breast-feeding you should supplement with vitamin D. Older people especially should take a vitamin D supplement. You should also take it if you eat no meat or oily fish, rarely go outdoors or cover up when you do.

The (RDA): 15mcg (USA) 5mcg (UK).

## Vitamin E

Vitamin E is a fat soluble vitamin which is needed to help maintain a lot of the tissues in your body especially the eyes, skin and liver. As it is an antioxidant vitamin, it stops your lungs getting damaged by polluted air and it also helps the production of red blood cells.

The richest sources of vitamin E are from plant oils such as soy, corn and olive oil as well as seeds, nuts, wheat germ, green leafy vegetables, egg yolk and olives.

The (RDA): 15mg (USA) 12mg (UK).

## Vitamin K (Phylloquinone)

Vitamin K is important in blood clotting to ensure that wounds heal properly; it's also needed to build strong bones.

Spinach, cereals, vegetable oils and broccoli are especially rich in it. You get small amounts in meats like pork and dairy produce such as cheese. But you also produce it yourself—in the friendly bacteria in your intestines.

The (RDA): 120mcg (USA) 75mcg (UK).

### Beta-carotene

An antioxidant vitamin. The antioxidant content gives orange and yellow fruits their color. Beta-carotene is turned into vitamin A in the body.

It's found in green and leafy vegetables such as spinach, carrots, red peppers and fruits such as melon, mango and apricots.

It is non-toxic in high doses as any excess passes out in the urine.

The (RDA): N/A (USA) 800mcg (UK).

### Co-enzyme Q10 (Co-Q10)

Co-enzyme Q10 (Co-Q10) is an antioxidant substance similar to a vitamin. It is manufactured in the body and is found in all body cells. Cells use it to provide energy that your body needs for cell growth and maintenance.

As a person ages, the production of Co-Q10 declines. Additionally certain medication—statins taken to lower cholesterol in particular, destroy Co-Q10. It is therefore beneficial to take a Co-Q10 supplement to make up for the shortfall.

Small amounts are found in many different foods. However, the highest concentration is found in organ meats: heart, liver and kidneys. It is also found in oily fish such as sardines and mackerel as well as peanuts and soy oil.

Co-Q10 has been used for many years by people with various cardiovascular conditions with positive results.

There is no (RDA) for Co-Q10.

# Chapter 22

## The Magic of Minerals

Every time you move your arms, blink your eyes turn your head—you are using minerals. Minerals are not produced by the body you get them from your food; therefore minerals are important for almost every body function. Calcium, magnesium and phosphorus are essential for bones and teeth. Nerve transmissions essential for brain and muscle actions depend on calcium, magnesium, sodium and potassium. Chromium is essential for controlling blood sugar levels. Zinc—an antioxidant mineral is essential as a free radical scavenger, also for body development as well as repair and renewal. Zinc and selenium—another antioxidant mineral supports your immune system.

There are two types of minerals—macro or essential minerals, and trace minerals which are needed in very tiny amounts by the body.

As mentioned above, they have three main functions:

- Building strong bones and teeth
- Controlling body fluids inside and outside cells
- Converting the food we eat into energy

The main macro or essential minerals are:

- Calcium
- Iron
- Magnesium
- Phosphorus
- Potassium
- Sodium
- Sulfur

The trace elements are:

- Boron
- Cobalt
- Copper
- Chromium

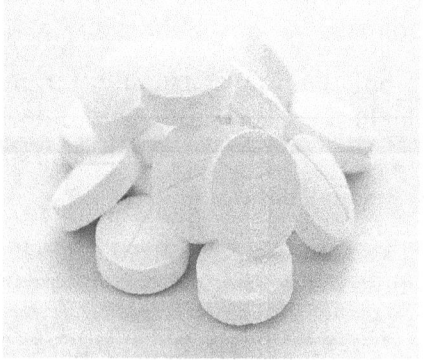

- Germanium
- Iodine
- Manganese
- Molybdenum
- Selenium
- Silicon
- Zinc

Let's have a look in more detail at the important things that minerals and trace elements do in the body.

**Boron**

This trace element assists the body in making the best use of fats, glucose, estrogen and other minerals such as copper, calcium and magnesium. It occurs widely in plants, oceans, rocks and soil and can be found in green vegetables, fruit and nuts.

There is no (RDA) for Boron.

**Calcium**

Calcium is one of the most crucial minerals we need. As well as building strong teeth and bones, it's important in regulating muscle contractions which includes the heart beat. It also ensures that your blood clots normally when you receive a cut. It is also an important mineral for maintaining the correct acid / alkaline balance

The main sources of calcium are milk, cheese and dairy products as well as green leafy vegetables such as cabbage broccoli, and okra (ladies' fingers). You also find it in soy beans, tofu, nuts, and bread made with fortified flour and fish such as sardines and pilchards when you eat the bones.

When taking calcium as a supplement, it is preferable to take it in a combination form of calcium and magnesium. Vitamin D should also be in the formula as it helps with the absorption of calcium. Also important is phosphorus, which works with calcium, boron, copper, and zinc (an antioxidant mineral).

Calcium supplements on their own can cause constipation in some people. Magnesium helps to counteract the constipation effect of the calcium. As separate supplements, take roughly half the amount of magnesium to what you are taking of calcium.

The (RDA): 1000mg (USA) 800mg (UK).

## Coral Calcium

As a high fat Western diet is acid forming which can lead to a condition called acidosis, coral calcium is naturally alkaline, so it can be really important for those people who want to keep their pH levels within the normal range. Coral Calcium is especially important for females as it helps support mineral levels in the female body, especially in regard to natural hormone fluctuations.

As well as supplying important calcium to the body, any formulation should also contain magnesium as these two minerals help each other. Vitamin D should be in the formula too as it aids in the absorption of calcium.

Middle-aged women as well as elderly men and women and those persons with a family history of osteoporosis, and white and Asian women between the ages of 11–35 can really benefit from an adequate calcium supplementation program.

There is no (RDA) for Coral Calcium.

## Chromium

Chromium helps to regulate insulin in the body and therefore has an effect on how much energy you get from your food. It helps to reduce food cravings and improves lifespan. It is also important for proper heart function.

This trace element can be found in soil, air, water, animals and plants. In food you get it from meat, whole grains, spices and lentils.

The (RDA): 35mcg (USA) 40mcg (UK).

## Cobalt

Cobalt forms part of the structure of vitamin B12 which I discussed earlier. It's found widely in the environment. Fish, nuts, leafy green vegetables such as spinach, broccoli and cereals containing oats are all good food sources.

Basically, to get enough cobalt you need to make sure you get enough vitamin B12.

There is no (RDA) for Cobalt.

## Copper

Copper is important in the production of both red and white blood cells. It also causes the release of iron to form hemoglobin, which is an iron-containing protein attached to red blood cells. This transports oxygen from the lungs to the rest of the body. Hemoglobin binds with oxygen in the lungs, which it then exchanges for carbon dioxide at the cellular level. It then transports the carbon dioxide back to the lungs to be exhaled.

Copper helps in child growth, the development of the brain and nervous system and for producing strong bones. In addition, it assists in maintaining healthy skin and hair color and is also used to diminish the effects of rheumatoid arthritis related inflammation.

It's found in nuts, shellfish and meat offal.

The (RDA): 900mcg (USA) 1mg (UK).

## Germanium

Many of the important herbs and medicinal plants traditionally used in healing, including ginseng, garlic, comfrey, and aloe vera, all contain substantial amounts of germanium. The therapeutic benefits of these herbs may be linked to the high amounts of germanium they contain.

Germanium also has antioxidant potential, and provides energy from carbohydrates in the diet. It's also found in a wide range of foods including beans, tomato juice, oysters and tuna, as well as those sources mentioned above.

Germanium comes in two forms—organic and inorganic. Inorganic germanium supplements have been withdrawn from sale because in this form they can damage the nervous system, liver and kidneys. The best organic supplements traditionally come from Japan where much of the research work has been done, particularly as a cancer preventative.

There is no (RDA) for Germanium.

## Iodine

Iodine helps make thyroid hormones which keep cells healthy and regulate your body's metabolic rate. It's found in seawater, seaweed,

Black Walnut, rocks and soil as well as cow's milk. Fish and shellfish are especially rich in it. But it's also found in plant foods such as cereals and grains but this depends to a large extent on the amount of iodine found in the soils where those plants are grown.

Every cell in the body needs iodine. Interestingly, if you put a small amount of this brown liquid on the back of your hand it will have disappeared within 24 hours. In fact it will have been absorbed by the body's cells which "line up" to get a "fix" of this important mineral.

Inflammation is one of the greatest threats to the human body. And is often a precursor to more serious health conditions developing. Iodine is very effective in reducing inflammation in the body and thus helping to protect you.

The (RDA): 150mcg (USA) 150mcg (UK).

**Iron**

This is another of those essential minerals just about everyone has heard of. It's vital in the production of red blood cells to move oxygen around the body. The traditional way to get iron into your system was through organ meat such as liver. But there are plenty of other sources such as beans, nuts, dried fruit, whole grains, breakfast cereals, soybean flour and most green leafed vegetables like water cress and curly kale.

A lot of people think that spinach is a good source but the problem is that spinach contains a substance which makes it harder for the body to absorb the iron from it. Strangely enough, both tea and coffee also contain substances which bind together with iron and make it more difficult for it to be absorbed. So cutting down on tea and coffee could boost your iron levels—and reduce your caffeine intake too.

On the other hand, eating foods rich in vitamin C at the same time as foods containing iron from non-meat sources might actually help with iron absorption. So fruit juice with your breakfast cereal or beans might prove beneficial.

Women who lose a lot of blood during their menstrual cycle may need iron supplements.

Women need more iron than men—around 14.8 mg as opposed to 8.7 mg for men.

The (RDA): 8mg (USA) 14mg (UK).

## Magnesium

Magnesium helps convert food to energy and makes sure that the parathyroid glands (which produce hormones to promote bone health) are working normally. It is also important for bones and teeth, as well as for the heart and nervous system. It is important for calcium uptake as well as being an anti-inflammatory mineral.

Magnesium can be obtained from nuts and green leafy vegetables as well as bread, meat, fish and dairy products.

The (RDA): 400mg (USA) 375mg (UK).

## Manganese

The trace element manganese helps activate over twenty enzymes in the body which assist in such things as digesting your food. It's often found in supplements. It is also important for healthy bone formation, cartilage, tissues and nerve function.

It occurs in bread, nuts, cereals and green vegetables such as peas and runner beans. Perhaps its main source for a lot of people is tea, drunk without milk.

The (RDA): 2.3mg (USA) 2mg (UK).

## Molybdenum

This is actually a heavy metal but as a trace element it's vital in activating those enzymes which produce and repair genetic material. It helps purge the body of waste protein by-products as well as detoxifying the body of free radicals, petroleum by-products and sulphites.

It is found in a lot of food, especially those vegetables which grow above ground such as peas, broccoli, spinach and cauliflower. It also occurs in nuts, tinned vegetables and oats.

The (RDA): 45mcg (USA) 50mcg (UK).

## Nickel

Nickel not only regulates the amount of iron in your body but it also plays a role in the production of red blood cells. It's important to note that one in ten people have an allergy to nickel so that if they come into contact with coins or jewelery containing it they may come out in a rash. The same can happen if you take supplements containing nickel and have an allergy.

Nickel is very widespread in the environment and lentils, nuts and oats are good sources.

There is no (RDA) for Nickel.

## Phosphorous

Phosphorous has a number of important functions such as building strong bones and teeth and helping to release food energy. It is a component of DNA and RNA, as well as helping to maintain the acid/alkaline balance of your body.

It's found in dairy foods, fish, poultry, bread, rice and oats.

The (RDA): 700mg (USA) 700mg (UK).

## Potassium

Potassium controls the balance of fluids in your body and it may also help to reduce blood pressure. Potassium makes it possible for essential nutrients to move into body cells, and for waste products to be eliminated from them. It is also involved in insulin secretion to control blood sugar which supplies energy to the body.

Fruit such as bananas are rich in it as are vegetables, pulses, nuts, seeds, milk, fish, shellfish, beef, chicken, turkey and bread.

The (RDA): 4700mg (USA) 2000mg (UK).

## Selenium

Selenium plays a key role in the function of your immune system, in the production of thyroid hormones and in reproduction. It's also a key player in the body's antioxidant defense system which prevents damage to cells and tissue. It is an antioxidant mineral and works with vitamin E.

Brazil nuts, bread, fish, meat and eggs are all rich sources.

The (RDA): 55mcg (USA) 55mcg (UK).

## Silicon

More well-known for the chips in our computers and other electrical gadgets, silicon helps maintain strong bones and helps keep your connective tissue healthy.

It is found in grains such as barley, oats and rice as well as in fruit and vegetables.

There is no (RDA) for Silicon.

**Sodium chloride**

Better known as salt, There has been a lot of discussion in the media and in government concerning the tendency for people to eat too much of it, especially in such things as processed foods, which often have very high levels added. Indeed most people do eat too much. But it's a vital substance in keeping the fluids in the body well balanced. And because it's a central ingredient of the juices in your stomach and intestines it helps you digest the food you eat.

Salt is found in low levels in virtually all foods. On average most people eat around 9.5 grams a day.

The (RDA): 1500mg (USA) 800mg (UK).

**Sulfur**

Sulfur's functions include the production of tissue such as cartilage. It is involved in many key body functions such as reducing inflammation, pain from arthritis and detoxification.

Sulfur is also a constituent of keratin and collagen which are found in hair, skin and nails. Therefore sulfur compounds are beneficial for these three areas.

One of the best forms of sulfur is the supplement MSM (methyl sulfonyl methane).

The therapeutic dose according to research into pain relief using MSM is a daily concentration between 1,500mg—3,000mg.

There is no (RDA)for Sulfur.

**Tin**

Very little research has been done on tin and its role in human health. One study showed psychological benefits of decreased depression and fatigue and an increase in positive mood and well being in some study recipients, while others experienced a reduction in headaches, asthma, insomnia and general levels of pain.

Tin is available in small amounts from virtually all fruits and vegetables. It is absorbed by plants from the soil. How much is found in food depends on the levels in the soil where the plants are grown.

There is no (RDA) for Tin.

**Vanadium**

Some interesting animal studies indicate that vanadium may help to normalize glucose levels, enhance athletic performance, and lower blood pressure. However, beneficial effects have yet to be conclusively proven in human studies.

Vanadium is a trace mineral that is essential for maintaining a healthy body. Vanadium is an opposite of molybdenum, which is another trace mineral, in that it works in tandem with it. Together, the two minerals help keep each other in check and provide several health benefits to humans.

In animal and human studies it has been found that vanadium helped to reduce blood sugar levels and also increased insulin sensitivity in those with type 1 and type 11 diabetes.

Food sources are seafood, cereals, mushrooms, parsley, corn, and soy.

There is no (RDA) for Vanadium.

**Zinc**

Zinc is an antioxidant mineral that helps make new cells and enzymes. It also functions with vitamins A and E to manufacture thyroid hormones.

It helps to process protein, fat and carbohydrate from foods and also with the healing of wounds.

Zinc is an important mineral in appetite control and a deficiency can cause a loss of taste and smell, thus creating a need for stronger tasting foods (which tend to be sweeter, saltier and more fattening.)

It's found in things like meat, shellfish, milk, dairy foods and cereals.

The (RDA): 11mg (USA) 15mg (UK).

Zinc Lozenges

Zinc is often combined with Echinacea and Licorice Root (as a natural sweetener) to treat the effects of a sore throat or other mouth infections. It also supplies excellent immune system support.

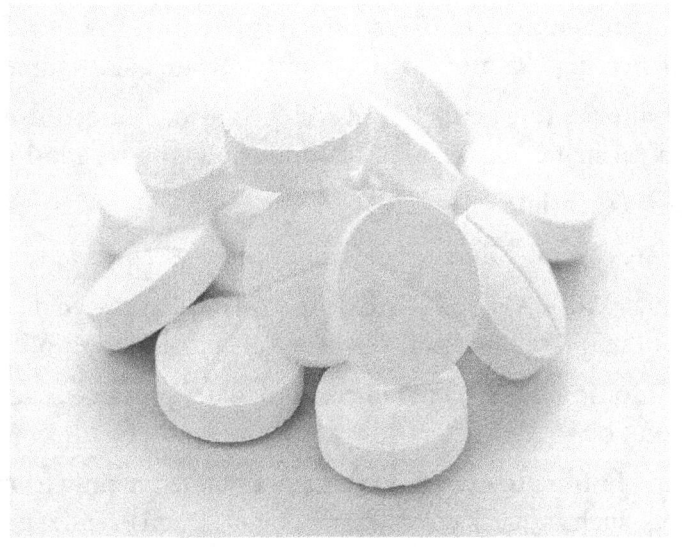

# Chapter 23

## Essential Fatty Acids (EFA's)

Essential Fatty Acids are so called because you have to get them from your diet—the body cannot make them itself. There are two essential fatty acids: omega-3 and omega-6. These two are the building blocks that make the twenty fatty acids that the body needs for good health.

### Omega-3 Essential Fatty Acids.

There are several different types of omega-3 essential fatty acids:

**Alpha Linolenic Acid (ALA)** good sources are: canola, flaxseed, rapeseed, soybeans, and walnuts.

**Eicosapentaenoic acid (EPA)** which is obtained from cold water, oily fish: herrings, salmon, sardines and tuna are good sources.

**Docosahexaenoic acid (DHA)** which is also obtained from cold water, oily fish: herrings, salmon, sardines and tuna are good sources.

### Omega-6 Essential Fatty Acids

There are several different types of omega-6 essential fatty acids:

**Linoleic Acid (LA)** good sources are corn oil, cottonseed oil, peanut oil, rice bran oil, safflower oil, Soybean oil and sunflower oil.

**Arachidonic acid (AA)** obtained from: dairy products, eggs, meat and peanut oil.

**Gamma Linolenic Acid (GLA)** this is obtained mainly from plant based oils, such as: black currant oil, borage oil, and evening primrose oil. In addition, most of these oils also contain some linoleic acid (LA).

Essential fatty acids are important for the manufacture of cell membranes as well as important hormones and neurotransmitters—chemical substances that pass messages between different cells which tell the body what to do.

They are also involved in the manufacture of prostaglandins in your body. These hormone-like substances help control many different activities. Some of these activities include such things as inflammation, pain, and unbelievably, some cause swelling and some reduce swelling. They are involved in allergic reactions, blood clotting and the manufacture of other hormones.

Prostaglandins also have a role to play in controlling blood pressure, heart and kidney function, body temperature in addition to being involved in the digestive system.

Being natural blood thinners, fatty acids help prevent blood clots, which can trigger a heart attack or stroke.

Arthritis and autoimmune diseases can be relieved by the natural anti-inflammatory compounds found in essential fatty acids.

If you experience skin problems or you have dull or brittle hair, if your nails split easily, or you have dandruff or eczema, then your diet could be lacking in essential fatty acids.

Essential Fatty Acids have an important role to play in good digestive and intestinal systems health. They help maintain cell stability in addition to increasing the thickness of cells lining the intestinal tract, as well as the villi which enhances the absorption of nutrients. All this leads to better digestion and improved health.

DHA—an omega-3 fatty acid is the most plentiful fat in the brain. It is important for ensuring that chemical messages pass effectively between the brain cells. Copious quantities of omega-3 fatty acids are also found in the retina of the eye.

Omega-3 fatty acids are also found in high concentrations in breast milk. Babies require it for their brain growth and vision development.

Low levels of essential fatty acids in the diet have been linked to vision problems, mood swings, memory loss and dementia.

So how much essential fatty acid should you take? It all depends on such factors as: what type of diet you have? The typical Western diet is very rich in omega-6 essential fatty acids which can cause a hormone imbalance leading to various health problems.

The ideal ratio is one portion of omega-3 to 5 portions of omega-6. In the typical Western diet which is high in saturated fat the ratio is often one portion of omega-3 to 20 portions of omega-6. To counteract this imbalance it might be a good idea to use the following formula. For every portion of omega 6, take 2 portions of omega-3. If you find it difficult to achieve this with your diet, then consider taking an omega-3 supplement. Incidentally, there is no Recommended Daily Allowance (RDA) for essential fatty acids. Men may need to take more than women. Also, if a person suffers from stress or health problems then more may be needed.

You may need to do your own experimentation to see how much you need. Have a look at your skin. If it is dry, then you should consider taking more omega-3. Skin that is well supplied with omega-3 feels supple to the touch. Remember in cold weather the skin can dry out necessitating an increased supply of omega-3.

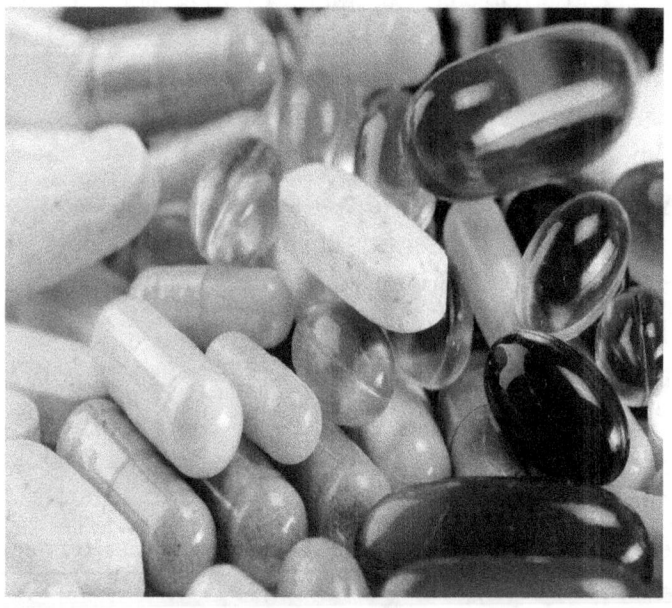

# Chapter 24

# Essential Fatty Acid Supplements

## Black Currant Oil

Black currant oil is a rich source of omega-3, linolenic essential fatty acid (EFA), alpha linolenic acid (ALA), and omega-6 gamma linoleic essential fatty acid (GLA), along with other important polyunsaturated fatty acids.

Fatty acids are involved in most body functions, from maintaining body temperature to providing a cushion for and protecting body tissue as well as protecting the nervous system and creating energy.

Interestingly, before the discovery of the benefits of black currant oil, the only other known sources of GLA were mother's milk and evening primrose oil.

## CLA

CLA, or conjugated linoleic acid, is a mixture of essential fatty acids that are important for maintaining healthy body functions.

CLA helps to sustain lean muscle mass as well as enhancing the burning of fat, which makes it a useful product in a weight-loss regime.

## DHA

DHA (docosahexaenoic acid) is an omega-3 fatty acid sourced from oily fish such as herring, mackerel, salmon, and sardines that is absorbed into the fatty perimeter of cells where it exerts its biochemical properties. DHA offers many benefits. It supports and protects the nervous system and supports brain and eye health as well as the health of the skin.

## Evening Primrose Oil

Evening Primrose is a plant that grows throughout the US and Europe. The plant grows close to the ground and the oil is found in the plants seeds. This oil is rich in gamma linolenic acid (GLA, an omega-6 essential fatty acid).

The oil is traditionally used to treat various skin conditions such as eczema and dermatitis and to alleviate breast tenderness from premenstrual syndrome (PMS).

Evening Primrose Oil seems to be more effective for the above conditions when taken with an omega-3 supplement from fish oil (derived from oily cold water fish such as salmon, tuna, mackerel and sardines) to create a healthy body balance.

Evening Primrose Oil is also used in the manufacture of some cosmetics and soap.

It is available as an oil or in capsule form. It should be kept out of direct sunlight and preferably stored in a refrigerator to prevent rancidity.

## Flax Seed Oil

The Flax plant is a blue, flowering plant that is grown in Ireland and the western Canadian prairies. No part of the plant is wasted. The inner stems contain fibers that are made into linen for use in the manufacture of bedding as well as clothes. The oil-rich seeds of the plant, known as flax seed oil or linseed oil, are used for cattle feed, in the paint industry, and as a rich source of omega-3 and -6 essential fatty acids for human consumption. These natural essential fatty acids are used for the general well-being and support of most body systems.

Flax Seed is considered to be one of nature's richest sources of alpha-linolenic acid (ALA)—(an omega-3 fatty acid)—as well as containing omega-6 essential fatty acids. In addition, flax seed oil contains B vitamins, potassium, lecithin, magnesium, fiber, protein, and zinc.

It also contains Lignans which are a type of fiber that is changed by "friendly bacteria" in the gut into compounds that fight against cancer.

## Krill Oil

Krill are tiny crustaceans that serve as a good food source for whales, seals, and other ocean mammals. They also provide a rich source of essential omega-3 fatty acids, including EPA and DHA.

Omega-3 essential fatty acids are important for cardiovascular and brain health as well as providing support for joints and the skin. Krill is a natural source of powerful antioxidant carotenoids.

Krill oil naturally contains phospholipids, which attach to omega-3 fatty acids, enhancing their absorption in the body. Phospholipids strengthen cell membranes as well as making them more elastic, which helps to keep toxins out and let nutrients and oxygen in.

**Omega-3 Essential Fatty Acids**

There are several different types of omega-3 essential fatty acids:

**Alpha Linolenic Acid (ALA)** good sources are: canola, flaxseed, rapeseed, soybeans, and walnuts.

**Eicosapentaenoic acid (EPA)** which is obtained from cold water, oily fish: herrings, salmon, sardines and tuna are good sources.

**Docosahexaenoic acid (DHA)** which is also obtained from cold water, oily fish: herrings, salmon, sardines and tuna are good sources.

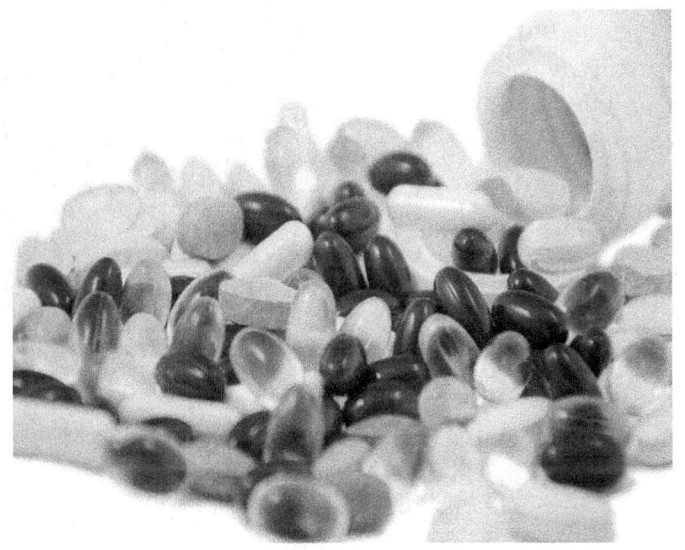

# Chapter 25

## Not a Vitamin, Not a Mineral, Not a Herb

### Acai Berry

The acai berry is an inch-long reddish, purple fruit. It comes from the acai palm tree which is native to the Brazilian Rainforest.

Acai Berry is a very powerful antioxidant which contains both anthocyanins and flavonoids.

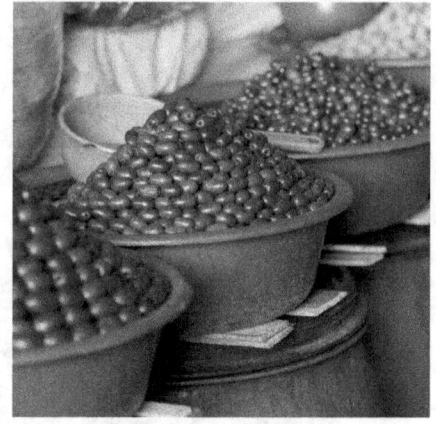

The word anthocyanin comes from two Greek words meaning "plant" and "blue." Anthocyanins provide the red, purple and blue color in fruits, vegetables, and flowers. Foods that are strongly colored such as acai, blueberries, red grapes and red wine, have very high anthocyanin activity.

Because of its high antioxidant activity, the acai berry is very effective at neutralizing the effects of free radical damage.

Currently there is a lot of marketing hype around acai berry with various claims of what it can do. It is heavily marketed for weight loss and is often combined with other herbal ingredients to make a combination product to treat various conditions in the human body. It is also marketed as an antioxidant to fight free radical damage.

In its native form, the fruit spoils very easily, so it is not available in your local supermarket, health food store, or on the Internet. However, it is often freeze dried for later use. This drying process does not appear to reduce the effectiveness of the fruit.

Acai oil is also used in some beauty and cosmetic products because of its high antioxidant activity. What makes it so useful for the cosmetics industry is that when it is processed and stored for long periods of time, the antioxidant potency does not degrade with age.

Acai oil is used in some facial and body creams, anti-aging skin treatments, shampoos and conditioners.

For human consumption it is available as a capsule or in liquid form.

## Activated Charcoal

Charcoal is highly absorbent. Activated Charcoal can help in cases of poisoning or severe diarrhea as it absorbs irritants and toxins in the digestive tract. It may also help lower cholesterol levels as well as relieving the effects of foul belching and severe smelly gas. An alternative to activated charcoal is to use bentonite clay.

## Alpha Lipoic Acid

Alpha lipoic acid is a very powerful antioxidant fatty acid which is found in every cell of the body. The body utilizes it to convert glucose (blood sugar) into energy for normal body functions.

Alpha lipoic acid is able to function in both water and fat, unlike the more common antioxidants vitamins C which functions in water and vitamin E which functions in fat.

A unique feature of Alpha Lipoic Acid is that it can recycle antioxidants such as vitamin C and glutathione after they have been expended. Meaning, they can be used again to fulfill body functions. Glutathione is an important antioxidant that assists the body in eliminating harmful substances. Alpha lipoic acid enhances the formation of glutathione.

Although the body manufactures Alpha Lipoic Acid, it is also found in brewer's yeast, broccoli, Brussels sprouts, organ meats, peas, rice bran and spinach.

Alpha Lipoic Acid is also intimately involved in brain function by crossing the blood brain barrier (a wall of structural cells and tiny blood vessels) to protect nerve and brain tissue from the effects of free radical damage.

Other uses for Alpha Lipoic Acid include: supporting the body after chemotherapy, dietary deficiencies, alcoholism, diabetes, kidney disease, Lyme disease, shingles and thyroid disorders.

Alpha Lipoic Acid is available as a supplement in capsule form, and in studies the daily amount that was best tolerated by the body, and to supply adequate amounts was 600mg, taken on an empty stomach.

## Apple Cider Vinegar

Excellent for vaginal yeast infections and external candida

conditions, it has good anti-fungal properties and can be added to warm bath water enabling a person to soak in it.

## Bentonite (montmorillonite) Clay

Bentonite clay is very quick acting as it has the ability to bind the stools together. It does this by binding irritants in the gastrointestinal tract. One option is to combine the bentonite clay with a small quantity of applesauce to make the clay more palatable. Applesauce contains pectin—another binding agent. Incidentally pectin is also used in jam making to make the fruit "set".

## Chinese Red Yeast Rice

Chinese Red Yeast Rice was first documented by the Tang Dynasty in 800AD. It is part of the daily diet of Chinese, Japanese and Asian communities to this day. Traditionally it is used as a food preservative, food colorant (it is responsible for the red color of Peking duck), as a spice, and an ingredient in rice wine.

Historical Medicinal uses include: a treatment for improving blood circulation, alleviating indigestion and diarrhea. In more recent time it has been used very effectively to lower cholesterol levels. This is due to it containing a family of monacolins (polyketides) with the ability to inhibit cholesterol synthesis and lower plasma cholesterol levels.

Traditionally the method used to make red yeast rice is to ferment the yeast naturally on a bed of non-glutinous whole rice kernels. This is rather a slow process which has been mechanized to produce dietary supplements containing the rice, yeast and Monascus fungus which is all contained in a gelatin capsule.

There are a number of natural compounds in Chinese Red Yeast Rice including: fatty acids and pigments in addition to monacolins (polyketides) mentioned above. The monacolins are believed to be the main component of the yeast's cholesterol lowering activity.

When combined with diet and lifestyle changes, Chinese Red Yeast Rice could be a good choice to lower cholesterol without side effects.

## Colloidal Silver

Colloidal silver has numerous uses and has been found to be effective against many surface and internal micro-organisms, viruses, protozoa, amoeba, fungi, parasites and yeasts. It works by in-activating the enzyme that is responsible for the multiplication of many of these invaders.

There are many different colloidal silver products on the market. You need to source one that contains 99.9 percent pure silver, without any additives, apart from water.

### Hoodia Gordonii

Hoodia is actually a succulent plant that grows in the semi-deserts of South Africa, Botswana, Namibia, and Angola. It grows in clumps of green upright stems which after five years produce a pale purple flower, at which time the plant can be harvested.

Interestingly, there are said to be more than 13 varieties of hoodia. But only hoodia gordonii has so far been identified as containing an active ingredient, a steroidal glycoside that has been named "p57".

Much of the marketing hype stems from stories of San Bushmen who live in the Kalahari Desert. These bushmen have taken hoodia for thousands of years to stave off hunger pangs and thirst whilst on long hunting trips. Today hoodia gordonii is sold as a weight loss product and is available as a capsule, powder, and tea or liquid.

### Lecithin

Lecithin is found in many food sources including cabbage, cauliflower, eggs, garbanzo beans, organic meat, seeds, soy beans, split peas and nuts. It is also manufactured by the body provided the correct nutrients are available for it to do so. Unfortunately this is not always the case with the average Western diet; therefore supplementation is almost always necessary. Supplements can be in either liquid or capsule form. Lecithin is non-toxic.

Lecithin is an important phospholipid which is needed and utilized by all body cells as well as the heart, liver and kidneys. As it is a fat itself, it adheres to cell and nerve linings, forming a slippery barrier to prevent cholesterol and other fats from sticking. This ensures that blood flows more freely.

When Lecithin breaks down body fats, it then transports these fats to the liver and helps convert them into usable energy.

## Methyl Sulfonyl Methane (MSM)

Methyl Sulfonyl Methane is a sulfur dietary supplement that starts life in the sea. Plankton in the sea release sulfur compounds which rise into the atmosphere where ultra violet light converts them into MSM and DMSO (dimethyl sulfoxide )—a precursor to MSM.

MSM and DMSO return to earth attached to rain droplets. MSM is found in grains, vegetables, fruits, meat and poultry.

MSM is an organic form of sulfur that is found in living tissues. MSM is the only dietary supplement that relieves allergies and arthritic conditions at the same time. In the structural system it is an excellent treatment for arthritis, muscle pains and bursitis. Additionally, it supports connective tissue such as ligaments, tendons, and muscle.

Sulfur is an important element in maintaining good health. But it is lacking in the Western diet. Therefore it would be worth considering as a preventative product.

## Morinda Citrifolia (Noni)

A native of the Polynesian Islands—Tahiti and Hawaii—Morinda Citrifolia (Noni) has been used by the Polynesians for over 2,000 years in a variety of treatments for various infections including: bacterial, viral, fungal and also for tumors. Additionally it has been used as a hypotensive, for anti-inflammatory conditions, and to support the immune system. Further uses include: boosting metabolism in a weight management program.

Morinda is available in capsules and also as a liquid. In liquid form the raw Morinda has a very bitter taste, so it is often sweetened with natural liquorice or glycerin.

## Proanthocyanidins

Often sold under the trade name Pycnogenol. Proanthocyanidins are powerful antioxidants obtained from grape seed and pine bark. They help prevent cell damage by quenching oxidative free radicals. This combination of antioxidant nutrients has been shown to be many times more powerful than vitamin C or E. Proanthocyanidins also improve the integrity of collagen fibers, in addition to strengthening tissues in the skin, blood vessels, muscles, cartilage and other connective tissue areas of the body.

## Tea Tree Oil

A native of Australia, Tea Tree Oil has many uses. It is highly prized for its antiseptic and anti-bacterial benefits. It is used to treat acne, athlete's foot, abscesses, boils, dandruff and Pyorrhea. It is also used to sterilize cuts.

### Algae and Seaweed:

## Chlorella

Chlorella is a single-celled green algae and contains over 19 amino acids. Of these eight are the essential ones in addition to beta carotene (which the body converts to vitamin A as needed). It also contains potassium and other important vitamins and minerals, plus enzymes.

Chlorella has natural antioxidant properties and as such, is a good detoxifier, cell enhancer and blood cleanser.

When taken as a liquid it eliminates body odors from the digestive tract, and is also an excellent mouth wash to eliminate bad breath.

## Irish Moss

Irish moss is a type of seaweed that soothes an irritated gastrointestinal tract. It is also used in hand and body lotion products to alleviate various skin conditions.

## Kelp

Kelp is a brown algae that comes from the sea. It responds to sunlight and takes in minerals and other nutrients from the water. It is an excellent source of iodine. Iodine is needed for proper functioning of the thyroid and pituitary glands.

The thyroid is responsible for maintaining metabolism and body temperature. In fact during stressful periods, the thyroid can work overtime to try and normalize body functions, therefore supplementing with kelp can be very beneficial for boosting energy.

A proper functioning metabolism is also important for maintaining weight control, which can sometimes be a problem when the body is under stress, and a person is susceptible to "binge eat" on comfort foods.

## Spirulina

Spirulina is a type of fresh-water blue-green algae composed of approximately 65-71 percent protein making it one of the richest known sources of vegetable protein. This protein is biologically complete, meaning it contains all 8 essential amino acids in their proper ratios.

Much of the protein in spirulina is in the form of biliprotein which has been pre-digested by the algae itself, making it 5 times easier to break down than either meat or soy protein. In fact, the digestibility of spirulina protein is rated 85 percent, compared to approximately 20 percent for beef protein.

This easy to digest type of protein is especially beneficial for those suffering from problems associated with excessive animal protein and refined foods intake: namely those with arthritis, cancer, diabetes, hypoglycemia, obesity, or similar degenerative conditions.

## Friendly Bacteria:
### Acidophilus

Provides friendly bacteria which normally resides in the intestines and is often destroyed through taking prescription antibiotics, using the birth pill or steroids. It can also be depleted though a dietary shortfall. These friendly bacteria can be replaced by taking a supplement in capsule form and/or through the diet.

### Bifidophilus

A probiotic supplement. Bifidophilus products contain living organisms from various strains of "friendly" bacteria to help replace depleted bacteria in the colon. They are necessary for proper immune function, and to help balance the digestive system.

Probiotics are very beneficial after taking a course of antibiotics. Antibiotics not only kill foreign invaders, but they kill "friendly" bacteria too.

### Probiotics

Probiotics are an essential part of good health as they keep "balance" in the body, as well as aiding the digestive, intestinal and immune systems. These "friendly" bacteria produce hydrogen peroxide which kills candida; thus in addition to its other health giving benefits it is a good supplement for anyone suffering from a candida yeast infection.

## Fiber

### Psyllium

An excellent source of dietary fiber, psyllium is gluten free and is therefore a useful fiber source for those suffering from celiac disease or a gluten intolerance.

It expands dramatically from the size of the original seeds and it is therefore essential to drink plenty of water with this product. Psyllium absorbs toxins from the intestinal tract and binds them to fecal matter for elimination.

As it is a bulking agent, it often gives a feeling of fullness and discourages a person from over eating. One of the main causes of constipation is a lack of fiber in the diet.

### Guar Gum

Is often used in fiber blends as it provides soluble digestible fiber. The body needs non-soluble as well as soluble fiber. Guar gum soaks toxins up like a sponge. It has a laxative effect, curbs appetite and is beneficial in lowering cholesterol.

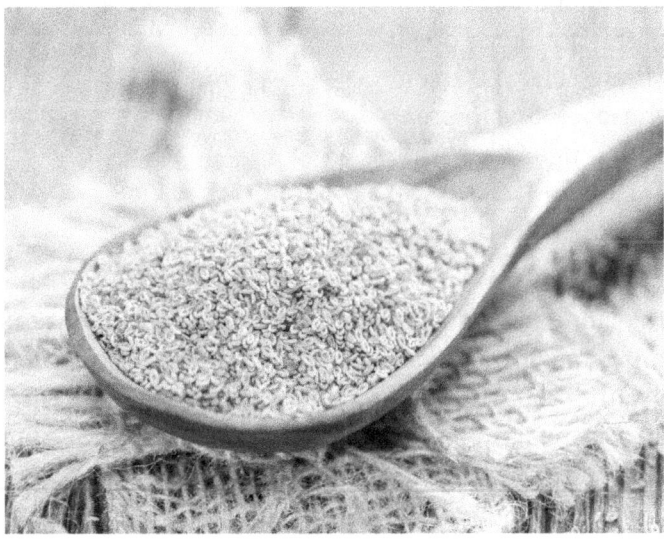

# Chapter 26

## Enzymes

We also need enzymes—all living things contain enzymes. Enzymes work as catalysts and produce energy. Enzymes are capable of performing these tasks because, unlike food proteins such as casein in egg albumin, gelatin, or soy protein, they are catalysts. This means that by their mere presence, and without being consumed in the process, enzymes can speed up chemical processes that would otherwise run very slowly, if at all. So in a nutshell, unlike vitamins and minerals, which are the building blocks of various body functions, enzymes are the body's workers—they make things happen. But very few people know about the vital role that enzymes play in maintaining a healthy body.

There are three broad classifications of enzymes: those that are contained naturally in the food itself, those that are manufactured by the body and assist in the breakdown and assimilation of food, and metabolic enzymes that provide chemical interactions within the body.

Each enzyme is designed to do a specific job. A protease enzyme (which breaks down protein) will not break down carbohydrates; likewise an enzyme whose job it is to break down milk sugar and milk protein (a job for lactase) will not break down fats (that is a job for lipase).

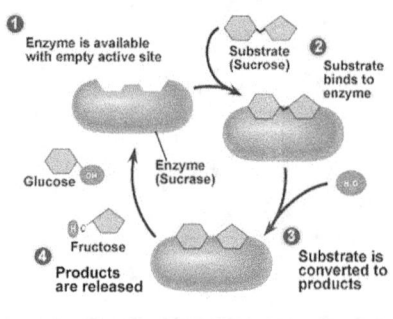

Nature planned for food enzymes to play an important role in the digestion of our food. Scientists say that digestive problems are a major health hazard in modern society. To explain the importance of enzymes is not easy, but my goal is to present an understanding of the role that enzymes play in keeping you healthy.

All raw, uncooked fruit, vegetables, meat, and poultry contain enzymes that will digest the food in which they are contained. The problem is that processing these foods destroys most of the enzymes. If food enzymes do some of the work, the body is not burdened with eliminating an accumulation of food it cannot assimilate.

Food allergies, gas and bloating, heartburn, and constipation or diarrhea are problems that can result from a lack of enzymes. Studies are gradually revealing that the resulting metabolic problems may be the direct cause of many chronic degenerative diseases.

To ensure that you get adequate enzymes, it is preferable to take enzyme supplements. These usually come in either enteric coated capsules (enteric meaning it will dissolve in the stomach or small intestine, and not before it gets to where it is supposed to work) or in tablet form.

Full spectrum enzyme supplements are available which means they contain enzymes that will assist in the breakdown of protein, carbohydrates, fats and starches. You may also see "proteolytic enzymes". These are in fact protease enzymes that break down proteins into their smallest elements. There are a large selection of enzyme supplements available, make sure you purchase one that is manufactured by a reputable supplier.

Sometimes an enzyme formula will contain hydrochloric acid (a stomach acid), which helps in the breakdown of foods in the stomach. As a person gets older, the body produces less of this acid, which can result in digestive problems and malabsorption of nutrients. If you have eaten a meal and feel as if you have a heavy weight in your stomach, then you may be lacking hydrochloric acid.

Here is a list of the main digestive enzymes and their function:

- **Alpha galactosidase** aids in the breakdown of complex carbohydrates commonly found in fruits and vegetables.
- **Amylase** (Mycozyme) digests starches.
- **Bile Salts** emulsify fats and prepare them for further digestion by the enzyme Lipase.
- **Cellulase** helps breakdown the cellular structure of plant fibers.
- **Glucoamylase** digests glucose sugars.
- **Invertase** aids in the breakdown of table sugar (sucrose).
- **Lactase** aids in the breakdown of milk sugar and milk protein.

- **Lipase** assists in the breakdown of dietary fats.

- **Malt Diastase** aids in the support of digestion and general nutrition.

- **Pancreatin** is produced by the pancreas to digest proteins, carbohydrates, and fats in the small intestine.

- **Papain** and **Bromelain** digest proteins.

- **Pepsin** is used for the digestion of proteins.

- **Peptidase** aids in the breakdown of proteins.

- **Protease** aids in the breakdown of proteins.

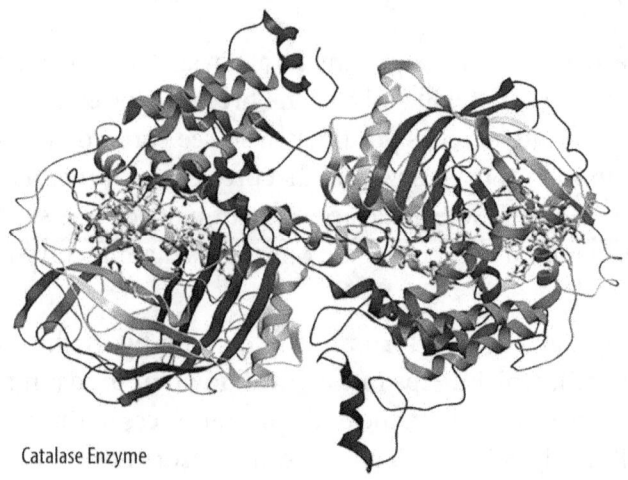

Catalase Enzyme

Catalase enzymes which are found in all living tissue (fruit, vegetables and animals) speed up a reaction within body cells which breaks down hydrogen peroxide, a toxic chemical, into two harmless substances—water and oxygen. This reaction is important to cells because hydrogen peroxide is produced as a byproduct of many normal body cellular reactions. If the cells did not break down the hydrogen peroxide, they would be poisoned and die.

# Chapter 27

# To Sum Up

A whole food lifestyle encourages good healthy eating and sound nutrition that makes sure your body is running at its best for years to come. Wholesome eating is an age old concept that has become lost in our high tech world where food is no longer natural, but is processed and manufactured.

But remember what I said about a "balanced diet". Everyone is different—some people need more of certain foods than others.

In addition, even wholesome food can be lacking in essential nutrients. A lot depends on how the crop is grown, how it is harvested, stored, distributed and cooked.

As soon as a plant is pulled from the soil its nutritional value starts to degrade.

A public awareness that there is often a lack of vital nutrients in food has led to a boom in the health food industry. Visit any health food store and you will find a vast array of vitamin and mineral supplements in addition to essential fatty acids, enzymes and various herbal products.

Maybe you feel that your diet contains all the necessary nutrients that you need for your particular lifestyle. However, if you have doubts, or are unsure, then you could always consider adding in nutritional insurance by supplementing your diet with high quality natural (not synthetic) dietary supplements. See page 115 for details of a supplier I have used for over 25 years.

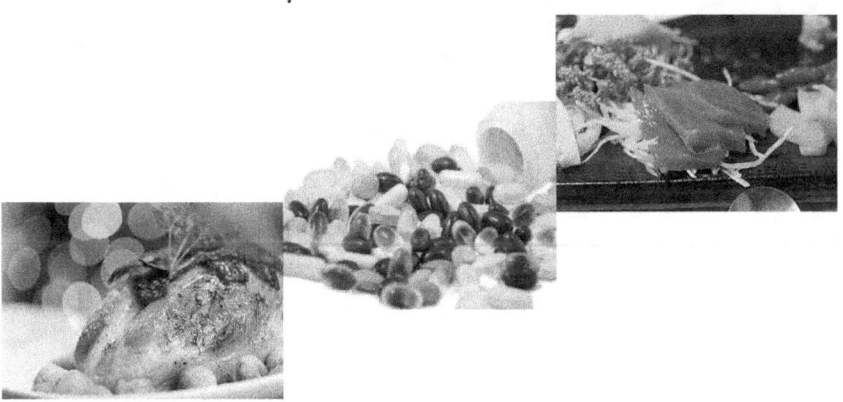

## About The Author

Brian B Jacques started in business at a young age, and over the ensuing years, he has developed several very successful businesses. But his main interest for the past 35 years has been in natural health research and publishing.

Brian has presented seminars worldwide on such diverse subjects as Health Related issues, Motivation and Personal Development. In addition he has written numerous books, newsletters and articles on these subjects.

His very popular series of Mini Health Books has circulated widely around the world, and many more titles are in preparation.

Brian is a highly motivated individual, so much so that in 1985 he received a UK Industrial Society award for his work in the Motivation and Personal Development fields.

Brian has the following mottos:

- If something does not work out for you, then don't give up, but keep trying, trying, trying until finally you succeed.
- Success or failure in any endeavor is in your own hands.

Brian was born in the UK and lives with his wife in Florida, USA.

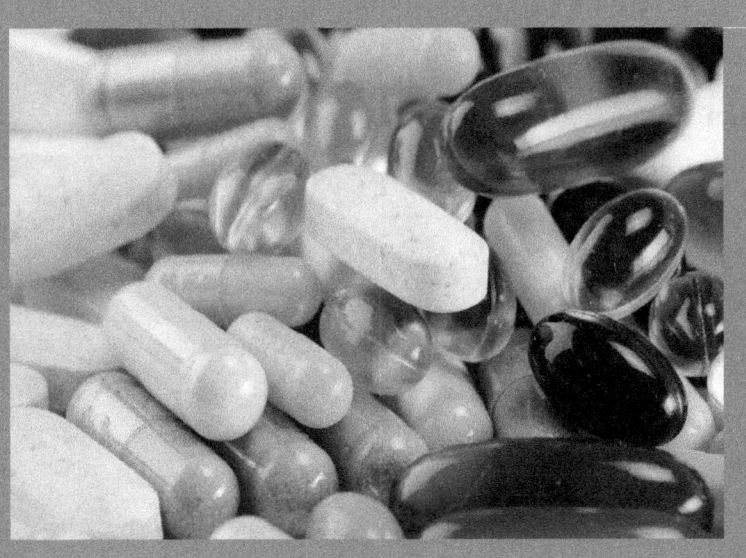

# Index